D1525000

Flu Action Plan

A Business Survival Guide

Flu Action Plan
A Business Survival Guide

Colum Murphy

WILEY

John Wiley & Sons (Asia) Pte. Ltd.

Other Wiley Editorial Offices
John Wiley & Sons, Inc., 111 River Street, Hoboken, NJ 07030, USA
John Wiley & Sons Ltd., The Atrium, Southern Gate, Chichester PO19 BSQ, England
John Wiley & Sons (Canada) Ltd., 5353 Dundas Street West, Suite 400, Toronto, Ontario M9B 6H8, Canada
John Wiley & Sons Australia Ltd., 42 McDougall Street, Milton, Queensland 4064, Australia
Wiley-VCH, Boschstrasse 12, D-69469 Weinheim Germany

Library of Congress Cataloging-in-Publication Data:

ISBN - 13 978-0470-82202-9
ISBN - 10 0-470-82202-3

Typeset in 11/14 point, ACaslon by Superskill
Printed in Singapore by Markono Print Media Pte Ltd
10 9 8 7 6 5 4 3 2 1

Contents

Acknowledgments   ix

Preface   xi

1   Know the Enemy   1
    Influenza: What It's Not   3
    Influenza: Under the Looking Glass   5
    Avian Influenza and H5N1   7
    Mutating Viruses: Shift and Drift   7
    H5N1 and Sars   12
    Avian Influenza: Only for the Birds?   13
    Migratory Birds: Vectors or Victims?   14
    Infiltrating Poultry   15
    Avian Influenza: Symptoms and Treatments   15
    A Question of Context   16

2   Learning from the Past   21
    Spanish Flu of 1918-19   23
    The Asian Flu: 1957-58   27
    Hong Kong Flu: 1968-69   29
    False Alarm: Swine Flu of 1976   30
    The Current Wave of Flu Anxiety   31
    Bird Flu Hits Hong Kong   32
    Sars   34
    The Lessons   35

3   Lessons from the Future?   41
    What Can Models Do?   43
    Human Behavior and Pandemics   46
    Looking to the Future   48

4   The Economic Impact of Pandemic Flu   51
    Economics of Pandemic Flu   52
    Overblown or Understated?   54
    Economic Impact of Pandemic Influenza   57
    Not Everyone is Convinced   59
    Conclusions   60

5   The Impact on Industry   63
    Different Industries, Different Impact   66
    Cross-cutting Infrastructure   70
    Hongkong Shanghai Banking Corp.   75
    Intel   77
    Hongkong Land   78
    Morgan Stanley Asia   80
    Cisco Systems Asia Pacific   82
    Conclusions   83
    The Impact of Sars on Cathay Pacific Airways   84
    Crisis Development   85
    Crisis Response   85
    Reassuring the Public   87
    Recovery from the Crisis   88
    Insurance Industry   89

6	So What's the Plan?	91
	Decisions, Decisions	95
	The Elements of a Pandemic Plan	99
	Tailoring the BCP	112
	Rehearsing and Activating the BCP	115
	WHO Global Pandemic Phases	116
	Conclusions	117
7	Disaster Averted?	121
	Down on the Farm	122
	Difficult Diagnoses	123
	In Tamiflu We Trust?	124
	The Quest for the Elusive Vaccine	126
	The Great Patent Debate	128
	Conclusion	133
	Resources	137
	Index	143

Acknowledgments

I would like to thank the following people for their kind help during the writing of this book:

To Arthur L. Reingold, MD, Professor and Head of the Division of Epidemiology, School of Public Health, UC Berkeley and Professor Stephen Chick of INSEAD for their invaluable suggestions and advice.

To Ryan Finstad and Emily Zylla, who provided excellent research and reporting assistance. Also, to Veronika Ruff.

To my "senpai," Jonathan Adams in Taipei, and Zach Coleman, for their stellar work and comments on earlier drafts.

To Pamela Ngai and the staff of the American Chamber of Commerce, Hong Kong for their efficient and courteous help.

To Terence Poon and the staff at the University of Hong Kong for arranging several rounds of interviews with HKU faculty.

To all the people — too numerous to mention here — who gave generously of their time to meet with me and share their insights with me. A special mention to Professor Malik Peiris and Dr. Gabriel Leung of HKU, and Craig Foster of Hill & Associates.

A word of appreciation to the corporations that willingly shared pandemic planning best practices and lessons learned from Sars: Cathay Pacific Airlines, HSBC, Intel, Cisco Systems Asia Pacific, Hongkong Land and Morgan Stanley Asia.

To the anonymous reviewers of earlier manuscripts, your comments are very much appreciated.

To those who helped out but were not at liberty to reveal their identities, a big thank you. Your "hands on" experiences of business continuity planning provided many valuable insights.

To my colleagues at the *Far Eastern Economic Review*: Hugo Restall, William MacNamara and especially Florence Lau.

Finally, to my editor C.J. Hwu at John Wiley & Sons in Singapore for her excellent suggestions and patient guidance.

Colum Murphy,
Hong Kong, SAR
June 2006

Preface

"Scaring people about avian influenza accomplishes nothing, because we're not asking people to do anything about it."

Richard Schabas, infectious disease expert
The Wall Street Journal Online, Jan. 13, 2005

London Calling

Barbara Newton* knew it was only a matter of time before she got "the call." It was early December 2005 and global media coverage of the avian influenza threat had reached a fever pitch. The disease had hopped, skipped and jumped its way from China through central Asia to Turkey — onto the doorstep of Europe.

The forty-something Australian took the late night call on her cell phone in her high-rise apartment in Hong Kong's Midlevels district. As human resources director for Asia with a European investment bank, she was used to getting calls from David Jenkins*, her boss in London, at the oddest hours. The two chatted regularly about payroll, recruitment and other personnel issues related to the bank's 3,000 Asia-based employees. But today was different.

"We need a plan, and we need it now," said Jenkins.

Headquarters had woken up to the threat of avian influenza.

Newton wasn't thrilled at the idea of dusting off the company's business continuity plan for pandemics, which had been developed during the 2003 outbreak of severe acute respiratory syndrome (Sars).

---

* Not their real names

She was certainly in no hurry to relive that experience. During the outbreak, bustling Hong Kong had become a ghost town. Almost immediately, the bank had slapped a moratorium on business travel. Anxiety among employees had been high, with some foreign executives demanding repatriation. Local staff complained bitterly of favoritism, and morale hit an all-time low.

Thankfully, Sars lasted less than six months, and it wasn't too long before business was back to normal. But Newton feared that an avian-flu pandemic could take an even greater toll on the company than Sars. She knew that developing and implementing a business continuity plan for bird flu would be far more demanding.

When her conversation with Jenkins ended, she dug out a version of the Sars plan she had stashed away in her home office, all the while cursing under her breath.

Feel The Fear?

Around the world, executives at companies like Newton's face the same dilemma. Should they draft a detailed plan for handling a pandemic and risk frightening employees and clients? Or should they ignore the threat and hope a flu pandemic won't happen? Since late 2005, more and more companies are deciding to take a proactive approach, even if that means they risk being seen as alarmists.

Conventional wisdom says that flu pandemics happen about once every 30 to 40 years. By this logic, the next pandemic is overdue. Yet the notion of a timetable for pandemics has been dismissed by others, who say that the last three major outbreaks — the Spanish flu of 1918 which claimed an estimated 40-60 million lives, the Asian flu of 1957-58 (two million dead) and the Hong Kong flu of 1968-69 (one million dead) — occurred at irregular intervals, with gaps of 39 years and 11 years. Critics of the "overdue" school of pandemic prediction say it is not the period of time since the last flu pandemic that matters. What is critical is whether the conditions are present for an outbreak now.

The World Health Organization (WHO) describes three conditions that would have to be satisfied for a pandemic to be triggered.[1] First, a brand-new, never-before-seen subtype of influenza must appear. Second, that virus must be able to make humans ill. And finally, it must be transmissible from one person to another. Of those three conditions, H5N1 — the current strain of avian influenza that has riveted the world — has satisfied the first two. But so far there is no evidence to suggest that the virus can be transmitted from human to human — and that may never happen.

What's At Stake?

The estimated deaths from a major flu pandemic have ranged from 1.4 million to a staggering 142 million.[2] The World Bank says the global economy could take an $800 billion hit.[3] Other economists say that even this figure is way too low.

Clearly, the experts can't agree on how serious a pandemic would be. But this much is clear: Even if the virus is "mild," the economic impact will be significant. That's because even a small outbreak could have an outsized psychological impact — especially since the public has been primed to panic by alarmist media reports. Sars, for example, showed that people's reactions aren't necessarily proportional to a disease's actual severity.

While a mild pandemic might not kill that many people (even though the "mild" Asian flu of 1957-58 still managed to claim two million lives), it could seriously damage the economy should the public overreact. Airlines, tourism, entertainment, retailing — industries that by nature demand close person-to-person contact — could be devastated by a mild flu as panicked customers opt to shut themselves off from society.

If more people fall ill with the flu-if there is a high "attack rate" — then absenteeism could affect productivity and supply chains could disintegrate. Many corporations that have developed pandemic plans have done so on the assumption that one in three of their employees will come down with the flu. Again, others say these estimations are too conservative. With a more lethal virus, international travel and trade could shudder to a standstill.

The psychological component of a pandemic is of particular significance to the corporate sector. Financial markets could crash. Public order could deteriorate, as hospitals become overwhelmed and citizens riot, demanding vaccines and antivirals.

H5N1: NOT ANOTHER Y2K

If these scenarios of doom and gloom sound familiar, it's probably because they are. In the late 1990s the world was caught in another frenzy of fear. That time the "virus" was the "millennium bug."

The Y2K bug was a problem written into computer software. In the early days of computer technology, disk and memory space were precious commodities so software code was trimmed down to the bare minimum in order to save memory. By eliminating the first two digits of the year in reference to dates and time — such that the year "1999" would be written as "99" — programmers devised ways to economize on the use of memory. What they failed to anticipate, however, is that the year "2000" would be written "00" — the same as the year "1900." As this realization spread and the date grew closer, experts began to speculate about the sweeping effects of this seemingly minute detail.

Around 1990 efforts to avert disaster began, and new software was developed to correct the problem. Still many feared that the Y2K bug, while a seemingly minor problem, could have disastrous consequences on the world economy as computers became snarled up around the globe. Reservations and records would be dated incorrectly, and some even speculated that worldwide calamity would result with power outages, satellite and communications blackouts sweeping the planet.

In 1998, Edward Yardeni, then-chief economist and managing director of Deutsche Morgan Grenfell, wrote in an op-ed piece in *The Wall Street Journal* that there was a 60% chance of a recession as a result of a Y2K meltdown.[4]

"The US may experience a $1 trillion drop in nominal GDP and a $1 trillion loss in stock market capitalization," he warned.

It never happened.

But in the late 1990s, who could tell between folly or wisdom? Most companies opted to be safe than sorry. An entire industry dedicated to fixing the bug emerged. In all, billions of dollars were spent trying to fix the problem. Some have placed the total figure spent on Y2K at between $1 trillion and $2 trillion dollars.[5] Of course, at the stroke of midnight, the world safely greeted the year 2000. The sky did not fall.

It would be easy to conclude that the Y2K mania was a product of alarmism. Many "experts" were seemingly left with egg on their faces. Likewise, the threat of pandemic flu may also turn out to be vastly inflated. Experts, government and health officials, business executives and journalists could all end up looking less than clever if a pandemic flu never materializes.

Yet it's impossible to know what would have happened on New Year's Eve, 1999, had the world not prepared so well. Some still argue that disaster was averted *because* the world was prodded into action — and there's no way to turn back the clock to see if they're right.

Moreover, a flu pandemic represents a very different type of threat. For one, there is no clear dateline for when a flu pandemic will strike. And unlike the millennium bug, there is ample historical evidence to show that flu pandemics can and do happen — always with devastating effects for humans.

About This Book

For years now, bird flu has been extensively reported in the global media. But outside of Asia, the disease did not truly take center stage until mid-2005.

That coverage has clearly begun to sink in for media-savvy executives. At a breakfast briefing in December 2005 organized by the American Chamber of Commerce (Amcham) in Hong Kong, participants asked fairly straightforward, nuts-and-bolts type questions: Is bird flu transmitted through the air or through droplets? How is avian influenza different from Sars? Should we stockpile Tamiflu?

But when AmCham organized a follow-up seminar in mid-February 2006, the executives posed different types of questions. They quizzed experts on how the corporate sector might be better armed for a pandemic: How should businesses that rely on heavy face-to-face contact with customers prepare? How should companies modify travel policies for pandemic situations? How should firms develop or modify their business continuity plans?

It's hard to say where most executives lie on this spectrum of awareness and knowledge of a flu pandemic threat.[6] Most realize that there is a danger. But how much of this awareness translates into knowledge, and how much of this knowledge is guiding continuity planning and corporate strategies?

Clearly some companies are more aware than others, and understanding of the threat posed by avian influenza remains patchy. The media are partly to blame. They have focused on tracking the spread of the deadly disease in birds and detailing the avian-related human deaths, repeatedly issuing disconcerting warnings, while offering few solutions.

To be fair, some of the larger news organizations have developed comprehensive websites that explain the disease. But they are the exceptions to the rule. Coverage of the disease devotes too much time on hyperbole and too little on lucid explanation of what avian flu is and how it might trigger a flu pandemic in humans. There's little straight talk on how it's contracted, how it's treated and how real the threat is. Nor is there much analysis of what is being done to prevent or mitigate flu pandemics. Even less attention is devoted to how the business community can prepare to deal with a pandemic.

This book aims to do that in clear and simple language. By examining pandemic flu from a corporate perspective, this book hopes to equip managers with the basic information and tools necessary for effective decision making.

The book's basic assumption is that a flu pandemic eventually will happen. This pandemic may not, however, be caused by H5N1, but by some other, completely different virus. So while the terms "avian flu" and "bird flu" will be the most commonly used, they are used as shorthand for pandemic flu, (not to be confused with seasonal flu, but more about that later).

The main message of this book is that by taking action now, companies can put policies in place that will protect their employees and their businesses. That threat may not be realized any time soon. But given the mounting evidence, the prudent approach would be to begin to take action now. Action that is founded on facts, not fear, is a company's best defense against the threat of a pandemic.

Endnotes

1   Avian influenza: assessing the pandemic threat, World Health Organization, January 2005, page 11

2   *Global Macroeconomic Consequences of Pandemic Influenza*, Warwick J. McKibbin and Alexandra A. Sidorenko, Lowy Institute for International Policy, February 2006

3   World Bank's Milan Brahmbhatt, senior economist with East Asia and Pacific Region, November 8, 2005

4   "Y2K: An Alarmist View," by Edward Yardeni, *The Wall Street Journal*, May 4, 1998

5   "Some Key Facts and Events in Y2K History," *Computerworld*, Jan. 3, 2000

6   For background information on awareness levels among corporations see: http://www.mercerhr.com/avianflu

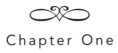

Chapter One

Know the Enemy

"I agree with the current concern on H5N1.
The reason being that if this were to become
pandemic it probably would be a pretty
nasty one."

Malik Peiris
Professor of Microbiology
University of Hong Kong

Malik Peiris does not look like the world's "hottest researcher." The title was bestowed to the University of Hong Kong microbiology professor by *Science Watch* magazine in 2005 in recognition of his ground-breaking research into Sars.[1] The 56-year old native of Sri Lanka exudes calm, yet little of what the clinical virologist has to say about avian flu is comforting.

Peiris has no doubt that a flu pandemic is on the way.

"The fact is a pandemic today will probably create a much greater impact in socioeconomic terms than 1968," he said, referring to the last flu pandemic, the Hong Kong flu, which claimed an estimated one million lives worldwide, including 34,000 in the United States. In 1968, air travel was in its infancy. Now, with millions of people flying across the planet on any given day, an infectious disease could spread very swiftly. Perhaps even more worrisome is the double-edged sword of the media. On the one hand, TV and newspaper coverage helps to keep the public informed about the latest developments and appropriate prevention measures. But the media can also stir the public's psyche in indeterminable ways. During Sars, panic pushed people to react in ways that, in hindsight, bore little or no correlation with the threat posed from the disease. In March 2003, working with a team of experts, Peiris pioneered research into Sars and made medical history when he identified the cause of the mysterious disease as being a novel coronavirus.

Mother Nature hates to be seen as predictable, and Peiris warned that there is no telling where the next pandemic might come from. "If you look at previous flu pandemics of 1957 and 1968, they did not come from a highly pathogenic avian influenza (HPAI). They came from some insignificant virus in birds."

Either way, the goal of a virus is to ensure its own survival by spreading to as many people as possible. The "enemy" surely will not be content to be a local player and confine its actions to one district, country or region (epidemic). Instead it will have designs to become a global star (pandemic), potentially affecting all people in all corners of the world. (Seasonal or annual flu is also global in nature. But in general, the term pandemic flu is used to describe a distinct type of influenza that arises from a marked shift in the genetic material of the influenza virus. The differences between seasonal and pandemic flu are discussed in greater detail below.)

Health officials and scientists like Peiris know they won't be able to prevent a flu pandemic working on their own. The public—including the business community—must be both informed and involved:

"We need to lift this [threat] to the broader community, to those who have not yet begun to understand the potential risks and consequences that a pandemic could have on every aspect of our society," US Secretary of Health and Human Services Michael Leavitt warned in December 2005.[2] "We need to have our schools, we need to have leaders of the economic community, we need to have the entire medical community, we need to have faith-based organizations [involved]," he said.

How can companies defend themselves? As in all wars, a good place to start is by knowing the enemy.

Influenza: What It's Not
Influenza is not the same as a cold. Table 1 describes how to tell the two apart. Differentiating between the two is not just a question of semantics. Confusion over these terms could have dangerous consequences when it comes to managing pandemic flu. When the next pandemic occurs, it is likely that among the employees of a large company, some people could be sick from pandemic flu, others from seasonal flu and still others from the common cold. During a pandemic crisis, the ability to weed out the colds from the influenzas will be crucial to ensure that precious resources are not wasted on harmless colds, and that a runny nose does not trigger flu hysteria.

But conflating colds and influenzas can have other implications. By associating a harmless cold with a potentially harmful flu, there is a risk of trivializing the latter. Even today with the increased awareness brought about by avian flu and the threat of a global pandemic, the perception remains among some in society that flu is not really such a big deal and therefore not worth worrying about too much.

Influenza should concern us. According to the United States Centers for Disease Control and Prevention (CDC), on average between 5% and 20% of the US population is infected each year by what is known as seasonal flu. More than 200,000 people are admitted to hospitals for flu-related complications, and 36,000 die

Table 1: Distinguishing Between a Cold and a Flu

	Cold	Flu
Symptoms		
Fever	Rare	Usual; high (100°F to 102°F (37° C-39° C); occasionally higher, especially in young children); lasts 3 to 4 days
Headache	Rare	Common
Aches, pains	Slight	Usual; often severe
Fatigue, weakness	Sometimes	Usual; can last up to 2 to 3 weeks
Extreme exhaustion	Never	Usual; at the beginning of the illness
Stuffy nose	Common	Sometimes
Sneezing	Usual	Sometimes
Sore throat	Common	Sometimes
Chest discomfort, cough	Mild to moderate; hacking cough	Common; can become severe
Treatment	Antihistamines Decongestant Nonsteroidal anti-inflammatory medicines	Antiviral medicines— see your doctor
Prevention	Wash your hands often. Avoid close contact with anyone with a cold	Annual vaccination; antiviral medicines— see your doctor
Complications	Sinus congestion Middle ear infection Asthma	Bronchitis, pneumonia; can be life-threatening

Courtesy: National Institute of Allergy and Infectious Diseases, Sept. 2005, www.niaid.nih.gov

from it annually.[3] Similar rates can be found in other countries and territories. For example, in Hong Kong—with a population of just under seven million people—around 1,000 people succumb to the flu every year.[4] As we shall see below, pandemic flu has the potential to be even nastier.

Influenza: Under the Looking Glass

Influenza is caused by a virus. The flu virus, like other viruses, is so small it can only be seen under a powerful microscope, but packs a punch potent enough to cause disease in creatures thousands of times its size. The flu virus normally hits the upper respiratory tract, i.e., the nose, throat and lungs. While there are three main families of flus—labeled A, B and C—the A family is of primary interest

Figure 1: The Influenza Virus

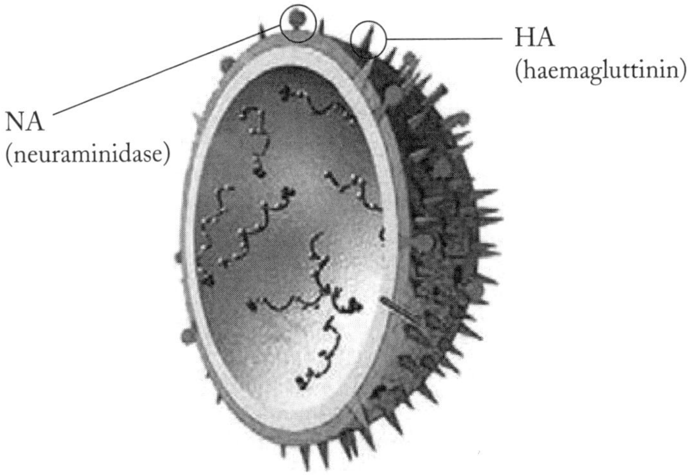

Source: WHO Influenza Handbook for Journalists, 2005

since this strain can cause death in animals and humans. H5N1 is a member of this family.

Influenza A virus is round or kidney shaped, and its surface is covered with a series of spikes. Its appearance brings to mind the rambutan fruit popular in Southeast Asia. As Figure 1 shows, there are two kinds of spikes, both of which are proteins: the hemagglutinin (HA) and the neuraminidase (NA).

"When we talk about H5N1 we are talking about a particular type of H and a particular type of N on the surface of the virus," explained Peiris. "These two proteins are very important in terms of our defenses. This is what our bodies' immune systems see and react against."

There are 16 types of HA, and nine types of NA proteins that can combine to form the avian flu viruses that are found commonly in birds, most frequently in wild or aquatic birds. The number of Influenza A subtype viruses that have caused serious illness in humans has so far been restricted to H1, H2, H3 of H and to the N1 and N2 subtypes of N. In addition, there are six other pieces of "genetic information" in the core of the influenza virus. Some of these genes function as the replication machinery for the virus. In considering an influenza virus, the whole package—outer proteins and inner genes—is important, noted Peiris.

The flu virus commandeers healthy cells, multiplies and moves on to do the same in other healthy cells, with devastating results for the victim. The workings of a virus have been compared to a gang of thieves, with one part of the gang specializing in breaking and entry (the HA) while the other (NA) is more adept at driving the getaway car. Some viruses are more pathogenic than others and can wreak enormous amounts of damage at staggering speed. Fluid and destroyed cells fill the victim's lungs, causing severe respiratory difficulties, which can result in death.

Avian Influenza and H5N1

There are at least 144 types of avian flu viruses. Most of them are harmless to humans. Many more are considered to be relatively harmless even to birds. And not all avian flus that jump the species barriers are lethal. In 1999, H9N2 was transmitted to humans, but it resulted only in mild illnesses. The same cannot be said for H5N1.

Within H5N1 there are many different subtypes, depending on the genetic information contained in the virus core. The differences may be minute, but could be significant when pharmaceutical companies try to develop effective vaccines.

To date, the strain causing the most trouble for scientists and public-health officials across Southeast Asia is the so-called Z genotype virus. Even within Southeast Asia, slight differences in the makeup of H5N1 viruses can be seen. The strain found in Vietnam and Indonesia, while clearly of the Z genotype family, are more like cousins to one another. These differences are not great enough to overcome one disturbing fact: that so far all strains of H5N1 can be transmitted from birds to humans. "The more this happens, the more chances of the virus adapting to a human pandemic situation," warned Peiris.

Mutating Viruses: Shift and Drift

Flu viruses are not static. If they were that would allow scientists to develop vaccines to stop them in their tracks. Instead, the influenza virus contorts and changes constantly, making it a moving target. The United States National Institute of Allergy and Infectious Disease (NIAID) counts Influenza A viruses among "the most changeable of viruses."[5]

There are two ways these viruses can transform—gradually or abruptly. After a virus attacks a cell, it leaves in pursuit of other cells to infect. Along the way, it continually replicates itself. However, Influenza A viruses are not very precise when it comes to copying themselves—the WHO even describes the viruses as "sloppy, capricious and promiscuous."[6] The result is that, little by little, through small incremental copying errors the virus changes. "This is antigenic drift—or minor changes antigenically—which allows the virus just that bit of space to escape the human immune response and give rise to another wave of human infection," Peiris explained. As a result, a drift variant of the virus emerges every two to three years.

The viruses can also change abruptly, in a process referred to as "antigenic shift." Scientists attributed the last two flu pandemics— the Asian flu of 1957-58 and the Hong Kong flu of 1968-69 to this. Because the process is more sudden, shifting can result in the creation of a completely new virus.

Peiris described a shift as a "lock, stock and barrel" change in the HA or NA. This can happen when a human flu virus picks up a completely different gene from an avian source. This phenomenon was first discovered by renowned flu expert Dr. Rob Webster more than four decades ago. Webster—who is currently a professor in the virology division of the infectious diseases department at St. Jude's Children's Research Hospital in Memphis, Tennessee— demonstrated how the Asian flu virus of 1957-58 was actually a hybrid of avian and human gene segments. Later it was confirmed that, of the total eight gene segments (i.e. the six genes found in the virus core plus the HA and NA proteins on the surface) of the Asian flu virus, three were avian in origin.[7] The same "shift" happened in the case of the Hong Kong flu of 1968-69.

It is precisely because of drift and shift of influenza viruses that there is so much concern about H5N1. If it were to change in some way, it might become efficient, allowing for easy transmission of the flu virus from one human to another.

Yet there is a difference between viruses that change as a result of drift or shift. The difference is largely related to the body's ability to fight against the newly formed virus. When a flu virus changes gradually over time, it retains many of the characteristics of previous strains. As a result, people who fell ill with earlier forms of the flu are more likely to have built up some immunity to the virus, which increases their chances of making a full recovery. In addition, because the new virus created through drifting is directly related to the old virus, developing a vaccine is a relatively straightforward process, although the formulae must be updated regularly (usually annually), in order to reflect the creeping changes in the virus. Antigenic drift is responsible for seasonal flu.

Even so, seasonal flu is hardly benign. According to the WHO,[8] annual flu epidemics affect between 5% and 15% of people worldwide every year, and result in a quarter to half a million deaths, mainly among elderly people.

When the new virus is a result of a shift in the makeup of the virus, the consequences can be much worse since there is no pre-existing immunity. This means, with current vaccine production methods, that sufficient quantities of an effective vaccine could take well over six months to develop. As NIAID pointed out, the appearance of antigenic shifts in influenza viruses "tends to coincide with severe flu epidemics or pandemics."[9]

With pandemic flu there really is no way of knowing what the death toll might be. The only point of reference is history. Pandemic flu has only occurred three times in the 20th century, each time with drastic consequences. With the arrival on the scene of a novel flu virus—natural immunity to which is nonexistent or at best, minimal—the proportion of people falling ill with the virus increases to between 20% to 50%. This compares to seasonal flu, the range of which, in the US, is between 5% and 50%. Table 2 examines the differences between seasonal and pandemic flu.

Table 2: Seasonal Flu and Pandemic Flu

Seasonal Flu	Pandemic Flu
Outbreaks follow predictable seasonal patterns; occurs annually, usually in winter, in temperate climates	Occurs rarely (three times in 20th century—last in 1968)
Usually some immunity built up from previous exposure	No previous exposure; little or no existing immunity
Healthy adults usually not at risk for serious complications; the very young, the elderly and those with certain underlying health conditions at increased risk for serious complications	Healthy people may be at increased risk for serious complications
Health systems can usually meet public and patient needs	Health systems may be overwhelmed
Vaccine developed based on known flu strains and available for annual flu season	Vaccine probably would not be available in the early stages of a pandemic
Adequate supplies of antivirals are usually available	Effective antivirals may be in limited supply
Average US deaths approximately 36,000 per annum	Number of deaths could be quite high (e.g., US 1918 death toll approximately 500,000)
Symptoms: fever, cough, runny nose, muscle pain. Deaths often caused by complications such as pneumonia	Symptoms may be more severe and complications more frequent
Generally causes modest impact on society (e.g., some school closing, encouragement of people who are sick to stay at home)	May cause major impact on society (e.g., widespread restrictions on travel, closings of schools and businesses, cancellation of large public gatherings)
Manageable impact on domestic and world economy	Potential for severe impact on domestic and world economy

Source: United States Department of Health & Human Services

H5N1 and Sars

Charged with drawing up a continuity plan, many executives, or at least those who experienced Sars in 2003, reach for the plan developed for dealing with that crisis. But there are several good reasons why they should not overly rely on their Sars plan when preparing for a flu pandemic.

"While there are useful lessons to be learned from Sars, the scale and potential impact are so radically different as to suggest a complete misapprehension of the risk," wrote Richard Martin of International Market Assessment Asia, a Sydney-based consulting firm that has issued a white paper on pandemic flu preparedness. "Sars is a starting point at best."[10]

It is easy to see why executives are tempted to make the comparison with Sars. In the first half of 2003, 26 countries reported outbreaks of the mysterious disease. In particular, many Asian economies—especially China, Hong Kong, Singapore and Taiwan—were badly hit by the previously unknown Sars. By the time a novel type of coronavirus was singled out as being the culprit, and health and government authorities had figured out effective ways to contain it, the disease had killed almost 800 people worldwide and cost the economies of affected nations hundreds of millions of dollars.

Yet this brush with a devastating pandemic pales in comparison to what pandemic flu could do. According to Dr. P.Y. Leung of Hong Kong's Center for Health Protection (CHP), one in 10 people who fell ill with Sars eventually died from the disease. This represents a high fatality rate, much higher than the past flu pandemics where rates of up to 5% were recorded. The difference, of course, is that the attack rate for pandemic flu is much greater. With anywhere between 20% and 50% of the population coming down with flu, and up to 5% of that number dying, the potential death toll in absolute figures is mind-boggling. In the case of H5N1 in humans, the fatality rate is a very alarming 55%.[11] Were H5N1 to trigger flu pandemic, that figure would be expected to drop to a range in line with past pandemics. As we shall see in subsequent chapters, most estimates of pandemic fatality are in the range of 1% to 2.5%. In addition, a flu pandemic, by definition, affects the entire world and not a selected few countries as was the case with Sars.

But perhaps the biggest difference is in the nature of the diseases. With Sars, patients displayed clear symptoms and they died in a matter of two or three days. A key symptom was the onset of fever. This allowed authorities to monitor people's temperatures as they traveled through airports and other check points. While doubt remains as to the overall effectiveness of such measures in containing the disease, at least it was technically feasible to do so. Furthermore, performing such checks no doubt had a positive psychological impact on a very fearful public.

In the case of pandemic flu, it will be much more difficult to identify flu carriers. Even though developing a high temperature is also one of the symptoms of flu, it is possible for an infected adult not to display symptoms and still be able to infect others. As the CDC explained:

"Healthy adults may be able to infect others one day before getting symptoms and up to five days after getting sick. Therefore, it is possible to give someone the flu before you know you are sick as well as while you are sick".[12]

Avian Influenza: Only For the Birds?

In the past, avian influenza was just that—a flu that infected birds. On the whole, avian influenzas rarely managed to break out of the avian world of birds and waterfowl such as ducks, geese and chickens. Occasionally other animals such as pigs became infected. CHP's Dr. P.Y. Leung considered avian flu in pigs to be "particularly worrisome" as pigs can act as a host for both avian and human influenzas, allowing them to act as a mixing vessel for both types of viruses.

That those infected with influenza virus can display clear signs that they are infected (symptomatic) or can appear healthy but still be infected (asymptomatic), has scientists and health experts worried, as it makes the identification of infected individuals and the control of outbreaks very tricky.

Of even greater concern is that H5N1 has managed to break through the species barrier. Avian influenza has been found in felines, including cats, tigers and leopards, and of course, it has also been found among humans.

Most avian influenzas are mild, but H5N1 falls into the particularly lethal highly pathogenic avian influenza (HPAI) category. HPAI was first defined as far back as 1878 in Italy, and the disease was previously referred to as "fowl plague." Since the outbreak of H5N1 bird flu in 1997, it has directly killed countless number of birds and has resulted in the culling of millions of others.

The WHO has characterized HPAI in poultry as being a:

> ... sudden onset of severe disease, rapid contagion and [with] a mortality rate that can approach 100% within 48 hours. In this form of the disease, the virus not only affects the respiratory tract, as in the mild form, but also invades multiple organs and tissues. The resulting massive internal hemorrhaging has earned it the lay name of "chicken Ebola."[13]

Migratory Birds: Vectors or Victims?

So how has bird flu managed to spread from its normal avian environment of ducks and waterfowl to infect domestic poultry— and humans—over such a wide geographic area?

For many, migratory birds are the clear villains in the spread of avian flu. The theory is that they come into contact with carriers of the disease such as other wild birds, ducks, geese, etc. The birds become infected but are asymptomatic. Then when migration season comes round, they fly off to far corners of the world where they infect other wild birds, and in some cases, domestic poultry. Often-controversial Hong Kong lawmaker Tommy Cheung even came up with a novel strategy to wipe out the bird flu threat: "Perhaps what we should do is give each person a gun and when we see a migrating bird, we can just shoot it down so Hong Kong would be a much safer place."[14]

Not everyone agrees. Mike Kilburn of the Hong Kong Bird Watching Society said that before blaming migratory birds, people should remember that wild birds are known to have been carriers of avian influenzas for centuries—without any serious negative effects on other species, and he pointed out that the disease only develops its lethal capacity when it infects domestic poultry.

Ornithologists like Kilburn said that "avian flu" is a misnomer and it should be renamed "poultry flu." Many point the finger at the poultry industry worldwide where millions of chickens are kept in such cramped conditions they literally end up walking in one another's contaminated feces, or being sprayed by other chickens' mucus when fellow coop dwellers sneeze (yes, chickens sneeze). Especially in Asia, where it is not unusual for overcrowded chicken coops to be built alongside human dwellings, this theory holds some appeal, casting doubt on the "blame it on the migratory birds" school of thought.

From an epidemiological perspective, the answer seems to lie somewhere in between. HKU's Peiris believed migratory birds to be guilty as charged, but that it was a matter of degree. "Without a doubt, the introduction of the virus to Romania, Turkey and Siberia is probably [traceable to] migratory birds, because all those viruses are very close to the virus causing the outbreak in Qinghai," he said, in reference to the Chinese province just northeast of Tibet and home to a serious bird-flu outbreak in the summer of 2005.

However, Peiris said that in areas where the virus is endemic, such as in Southeast Asia, the bulk of the transmission of the disease and its subsequent perpetration, is a result of poultry movement. In other words, migratory birds may introduce it, but it is spread as large volumes of chickens are moved around in the region either as part of the small-scale or industrial-scale trade in poultry.

Infiltrating Poultry

Once the disease enters domestic poultry, it begins to take on a more significant threat to humans. This is because hundreds of millions of people around the world make their livelihoods from rearing chickens. So far, nearly all cases where bird flu has been transmitted to humans has involved the victim coming into close proximity to live poultry through poultry farming, or in the wet markets that form the backbone of food retailing in many countries, or through direct involvement in the culling of infected chickens.

Incidentally, eating cooked chicken is not considered risky, if care is taken to ensure that the chicken is properly cooked at appropriate heat levels. The WHO's International Food Safety Authorities Network says cooking at 70 degrees Celsius will inactivate the H5N1 virus. Freezing and refrigeration will not kill the virus, it warns.[15]

Avian Influenza: Symptoms and Treatments

What happens when a human catches bird flu from poultry? The symptoms include those typically associated with a flu—fever, cough, sore throat and aching muscles. In addition, bird-flu symptoms can include eye infection, pneumonia and other severe respiratory conditions.

In the absence of a vaccine, the only other medical option available is to take antiviral drugs called neuraminidase inhibitors. The most famous of these is oseltamivir, commonly referred to by its brand name, Tamiflu. A less well-known alternative is zanamivir, which is commercially known as Relenza. To be effective, both of these drugs need to be administered within 48 hours after the onset of symptoms.

There is growing evidence to suggest that Tamiflu and Relenza may not be the bird-flu panacea they are widely thought to be.

With regard to vaccines, there are several problems associated with the effective development and manufacturing of appropriate vaccines. Chapter Seven looks at the issue of vaccines in greater detail.

Antibiotics offer no protection from avian influenza, but they are effective against pneumonia, and other secondary bacterial infections that may result from the body's weakened state.

A Question of Context

Are we paying too much attention to avian influenza and its potential to trigger a flu pandemic? The amount of money that has been earmarked to deal with the problem is significant. The United States Congress agreed to allocate more than $3 billion in late 2005.[16] In January 2006, international donors pledged another $1.9 billion.[17] Yet the number of deaths from avian flu remains in the low hundreds. How can we justify this in a world where countless other diseases ravage populations and cause far more pain and hardship?

Shigeru Omi, the WHO's regional director for the Western Pacific region, saw global health challenges as falling into one of three categories: emerging and re-emerging infectious communicable diseases; noncommunicable diseases including diabetes or smoking-related illnesses (WHO estimates that 17 million people die prematurely from chronic diseases every year[18]); and challenges relating to the healthcare system.

Avian flu and pandemic flu fall into the first category—a category it shares with diseases such as HIV/AIDS. The WHO says that "despite measures designed to prevent the HIV/AIDS virus from spreading, five million people worldwide were needlessly infected last year, [2005] adding to the 40 million already living with the virus." Globally, a total of 3.1 million people died from HIV/AIDS in 2005. In Asia, an estimated eight million are infected with HIV/AIDS, including 650,000 people in China. Yet only one in seven Asians with HIV/AIDS had access to antiretroviral therapy, important treatment for those infected.[19]

On HIV/AIDS Dr. Omi said: "We know what works and what doesn't. So why has the necessary action to prevent the virus from spreading not been taken? Why is the epidemic still growing and not reversing?"

While companies are starting to wake up to the long-term threats of chronic diseases by implementing no-smoking rules and other policies to promote health, few have done anything to incorporate HIV/AIDS into their business planning. In a survey released in January 2006, the Global Health Initiative of the World Economic Forum said that only 18% of 11,000 companies polled had policies addressing the issues of discrimination in promotion, pay or benefits based on HIV status.[20] But as the same survey pointed out, there is increased anxiety among business leaders that HIV/AIDS will affect their operations over the course of the next five years, with 46% of companies expressing concern (up from 37% one year earlier).

The question is: should governments and companies pay attention to a pandemic flu that might never happen?

Dr. Omi said yes. "Potentially it can be even more dangerous [than HIV/AIDS]."

Economist Jeffrey Sachs, Director of the Earth Institute at Columbia University agreed that the attention is merited.

"A flu pandemic is a very real possibility, with potentially devastating consequences if it occurs," he writes in an email response to questions. "And as in many other areas of disease control, e.g., AIDS, malaria, etc., attention to a single disease such as avian flu will strengthen the overall health system, in terms of public knowledge, epidemic surveillance, medical research and on-the-ground delivery of preventative and therapeutic measures."

But perhaps the most compelling evidence comes from history. Most fears of a future flu pandemic are grounded in past experiences, particularly the 1918-19 Spanish flu virus which claimed an estimated 40 to 60 million lives worldwide. Chapter 2 poses the question: What lessons can be learned from the past?

Endnotes

1   Thomson Scientific Names "Hottest" Researchers, company press release, March 24, 2005

2   Michael Leavitt, US Secretary of Health and Human Services in a Dec. 5, 2005 summit on pandemic preparedness in Washington, DC.

3   see http://www.cdc.gov/flu/keyfacts.htm

4   Dr. P.Y. Leung, Controller of Hong Kong's Center for Health Protection. Presentation, November 2005

5   See http://www3.niaid.nih.gov/news/focuson/flu/research/primer/

6   "Avian influenza: assessing the pandemic threat," *WHO*, January 2005, page 10

7   "Scientists Race To Head Off Lethal Potential of Avian Flu," David Brown, *The Washington Post*, August 23, 2005

8   "WHO Handbook for Journalists: Influenza Pandemic," *WHO*, December 2005, page 2

9   See http://www3.niaid.nih.gov/news/focuson/flu/research/primer/

10   See http://www.imaasia.com/BirdFluIMA%20Asia_Jan06.pdf

11 See http://www.who.int/csr/disease/avian_influenza/country/cases_table_2006_04_21/en/index.html

12 See http://www.cdc.gov/flu/symptoms.htm

13 See http://www.who.int/mediacentre/factsheets/avian_influenza/en/index.html

14 As reported by the Associated Press, Oct. 28, 2005

15 See http://www.who.int/foodsafety/fs_management/No_02_Avianinfluenza_Dec04_en.pdf

16 See 2005 Legislative Summary: Pandemic Flu Preparedness, by Kate Schuler, Dec. 30, 2005 in *CQ Weekly*

17 "See Donors Pledge \$1.9 Billion to Fight Avian Flu in Developing Nations," by Shai Oster, *The Wall Street Journal*, Jan. 19, 2006

18 See http://www.who.int/mediacentre/news/releases/2005/pr47/en/index.html

19 See http://www.wpro.who.int/media_centre/press_releases/pr_20051129.htm

20 See http://www.weforum.org/site/homepublic.nsf/Content/Global+Health+Initiative%5CGHI+Global+Business+Survey

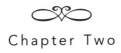

Chapter Two

Learning from the Past

"...people in good health were all of a
sudden attacked by violent heats in the head,
and redness and inflammation in the eyes,
the inward parts, such as the throat or
tongue, becoming bloody and emitting an
unnatural and fetid breath."[1]

Thucydides,
The History of the Peloponnesian War

Pandemics have been around probably as long as humanity. In what is thought to be the first recorded pandemic, the Greek aristocrat and historian Thucydides detailed the grizzly symptoms of the mysterious disease which ravaged Athens around 430 B.C., killing one in three citizens.

Author Mary Ellen Snodgrass has meticulously logged thousands of pandemics and epidemics, from the bacterial traces of the infectious skin disease yaws discovered in the remains of prehistoric man, to the present century and the emergence of new diseases such as Sars.[2]

Most pandemics have been forgotten. Others, like the bubonic plague, retain their ghastly notoriety. Also known as the Black Death, this infectious disease was caused by bacteria found in rodents and spread to humans by fleas. Twenty-four million people in Europe died between 1347 and 1351. The last pandemic of bubonic plague originated in Hong Kong in the mid-1890s.

Cholera was one of the most feared diseases of the 19th century, and still poses a major problem in parts of Africa and Asia. In India, where it first emerged in epidemic form in 1817, 25 million people died from the disease during the 18th century and first quarter of the 19th. Cholera arrived in the United Kingdom in 1831, and by the end of the 19th century, had claimed the lives of an estimated 130,000 Britons.[3]

Of the more than 70 outbreaks of influenza chronicled by Snodgrass, most were epidemics, or localized outbreaks. But at least four flu pandemics, or global outbreaks, occurred in the 19th century, and possibly as many as six in the 18th century.

Few meaningful records exist from these earlier flu pandemics. However, that changed in the 20th century, when the horrific Spanish flu of 1918-19 resulted in a dramatic improvement in the keeping of medical records.

* * * * * * * * * * * * * *

Thirty miles off the coast of Massachusetts, from his retirement home on the island of Nantucket, historian Alfred Crosby keeps a watchful eye on the evolution of bird flu. Three decades ago the professor emeritus at the University of Texas in Austin wrote *America's Forgotten Pandemic: The Influenza of 1918*.[4] The book is still considered to be the definitive account of the Spanish flu.

According to Crosby, there are many lessons to learn from history: "Studying the last killing pandemic might well tell us something useful about the next," he wrote in an email interview. "[And] such a study might also tell us about how societies act during sieges."

The Spanish flu, as well as the Asian and Hong Kong influenzas (the two other flu pandemics of the last century), remind us how lethal flu pandemics can be. Yet more than just scaring us, past pandemics offer critical clues to help us better plan for future ones, and can help us answer vital questions such as: What was the epidemiological evolution of previous flu pandemics? How was the disease distributed among different age groups? Was quarantine an effective way of containing the spread of the disease? Public-health officials are not the only ones that can benefit from studying past flu pandemics. Business leaders, too, can gain from the exercise. How did flu pandemics affect the economies? How were markets affected? For modern businesses, the Sars crisis provides plenty of case studies from which to learn.

Finally, pandemics that never materialize are also worth examining, if only to drive home the message that appropriate action, not panic, must always guide our actions.

Spanish Flu of 1918-19

The most frequently evoked example of a killer flu pandemic is the Spanish flu of 1918-19. It certainly offers a dramatic wake-up call for those tempted to downplay the avian influenza threat. It is sometimes called the Purple Plague in reference to the color some victims displayed right before they died. As *New York Times* science reporter Gina Kolata so poignantly described in her book, *Flu*, the Spanish flu was vicious, attacking in one of two ways:

> *"Some (victims) almost immediately became deathly ill, unable to get enough oxygen because their lungs had filled with fluid. They died in days, even hours, delirious with a high fever, gasping for breath, lapsing at last into unconsciousness. In others, the illness began as an ordinary flu, with chills, fever, and muscle aches, but*

no untoward symptoms. By the fourth or fifth day of the illness, however, bacteria would swarm into their injured lungs and they would develop pneumonia that would either kill them or lead to a long period of convalescence."[5]

Spanish flu was later identified as the H1N1 virus, which took the lives of as many as 600,000 people in the United States alone, and an estimated 40 to 60 million people around the world. That is more than the number of people killed in World War I, which was in full swing when the flu embarked on its world tour. The war ended on November 11, 1918—Armistice Day—several months before the deadly virus began to fizzle out.

Despite its name, the Spanish flu did not originate on the Iberian Peninsula. The most deadly flu pandemic in living memory was named after Spain simply because that is where the first reports of the disease emerged. During World War I, both the British and American media were heavily censored since revealing any weakness, natural or military, could present the Germans with a psychological advantage.

This inability, or unwillingness, to disseminate information freely would exact a price. By stamping it "Top Secret," authorities had given the other enemy, the flu, a helping hand. In any future flu pandemic, open and free communication will play a pivotal role in stemming the spread of infections.

If the virus did not originate in Iberia, then where did it come from? The most probable theory, and the one featured by author John Barry in his book *The Great Influenza*, traces the origin to Haskell County, Kansas.[6] In early spring of 1918, a group of young army officers based at Camp Funston (also in Kansas) were thought to have contracted the virus while on home leave. On their return to base, they spread the flu to other officers. Frequent exchange of soldiers between bases meant the infection was soon spreading to other camps along the east coast of the US. The large numbers of men living in cramped quarters only served to facilitate transmission of the illness. When troops were mobilized from the US and sent to the war front in Western Europe, the virus also made the trip across the Atlantic. By early April it had made its way to Brest, a shipping hub in northwest France through which a large number of American troops transited en route to the front. The disease then spread from the confines of US troop facilities and infiltrated the quarters of French and British soldiers. By the end of April, Barry wrote, the flu virus "exploded." It even reached other continents, with reports of an outbreak in Bombay, India as early as the end of May, and from Shanghai around the same time.

From France, the flu spread to Italy, Spain, Portugal and Greece. By June it had reached Germany; and Denmark and Norway by July. Pandemic flu spreads in waves, and this was still the first wave. Although the flu was severely debilitating, at this stage it had yet to turn lethal. Between the beginning of June and the start of August, out of a total of two million troops deployed in France, records show that one tenth had become so ill they were unable to report for duty. Coming at the height of battle, the timing could not have been worse.

From there, the situation deteriorated even further. By early fall, the virus had transformed into a killer. By then, it had been reintroduced to the US, prompting Congress to approve a $1 million appropriation to fight the disease. Yet this would not be enough to stem the illness and death that followed during the second and third waves of the flu, until its retreat in spring of 1919.

In particular, the east coast of the US was hard-hit. Philadelphia bore the brunt, something many attribute to the incompetent handling of the outbreak by city officials. Boston and New York also came under attack. Over the following weeks, the disease spread westward to California. The first wave peaked in the

October-November period. At the outset, Spanish flu behaved like a seasonal flu, affecting children and the elderly. But when it became more virulent, it changed its tack and began to go for young people in their prime.

The rest of the world did not escape the effects of the Spanish flu. From Uruguay (2,050 dead) to Afghanistan (320,000 dead); from Italy (390,000 dead) to India (18.5 million dead), almost no country was left untouched.[7]

But is the Spanish flu an appropriate pandemic against which to benchmark a future flu? Some say no and point to circumstances in 1918 they say were especially conducive to the spread of flu. These included the overcrowded and filthy conditions of the war trenches, and the unusually high traffic in army personnel moving back and forth between the US, the United Kingdom and continental Europe. Both of these factors exacerbated the spread of killer germs, they say. But today, the squalor and population density that can be found in the mega-cities of the developing world is as startling as any World War I trench. And the countless number of people that travel across continents on airplanes on a daily basis surely poses a far greater risk for the propagation of disease than the troop deployments of World War I.

Others argue that medical science in 1918 was extremely unsophisticated when compared with today. At that time, doctors did not even know what caused influenza—a virus or bacteria. There was no effective vaccine developed—and one would not be until the 1930s. Antiviral drugs were unavailable. Even the most basic hygiene and safety measures—such as the use of face masks—had only just begun to gain a foothold at the time.

This is why some consider the Spanish flu to be an anomaly. The WHO states:

"...because the 1918 pandemic was the single most devastating infectious disease outbreak ever recorded, WHO does not feel it is appropriate to project future pandemic numbers based on such an exceptional event." [8]

Yet it would be unwise to entirely dismiss the Spanish flu as a benchmark for future pandemics, not least because it is always prudent to examine the worst case scenarios when planning for future catastrophes. In this respect, the Spanish flu certainly fits the part, representing many public-health officials' worst pandemic flu nightmare. What's more, if a pandemic with the same potency were to strike today, it could claim the lives of many more millions of people than the number killed in 1918, just by virtue of the growth in the overall population of the planet which has tripled in the past century.

The Asian Flu: 1957-58

The second flu pandemic of the 20th century struck in 1957. Known as the Asian flu, the virus was H2N2 in its makeup. The pandemic shared some of the broader characteristics of the Spanish flu. For example, it also came in waves. The pandemic first emerged in China in February 1957. In May, reports of flu outbreaks in Hong Kong and Singapore were received by the WHO. By the summer the virus had arrived in the US. By the time it petered out in 1958, Asian flu had killed 70,000 Americans. Worldwide, that figure reached two million. [9]

Again, the first wave of this flu pandemic was relatively mild. In the US, it was only in early autumn, when children returned to school after the summer vacation, that infections exploded. The worst period for flu and pneumonia-related deaths was September to December of 1957. The second wave struck in January and February of 1958. This time elderly people were hardest hit.

The evolution of the Spanish flu was different from that of the Asian flu. The Spanish flu is thought to have been an avian influenza that leaped from chickens to humans. In contrast, the Asian flu was a re-assortment among existing human influenza viruses.

The number of deaths arising from Asian flu was a fraction of the Spanish flu. This was because the 1957-58 pandemic was caused by a milder virus. Other factors, no doubt, played a role. For instance, great advances had been made in medicine and public hygiene since 1918. Chief among these were the significant strides that had been achieved in vaccine development. By August 1957, just six months after initial reports of the flu, a vaccine was developed and available for distribution. True, vaccine production was on a limited scale, and then only in the US. Other developed countries, including the United Kingdom, followed suit two or three months later. As the WHO observed:

> "Countries with domestic capacity were able to produce enough vaccine, early enough, to protect priority groups only. No country had sufficient production capacity to cover its entire population, much less to export vaccines elsewhere..."[10]

Also, by the time of the Asian flu, antibiotics had been developed that were effective against bacterial infections. This is important since bacterial pneumonia has always been a close and deadly companion of influenza. In addition, international cooperation in the field of medicine was in full swing by 1957. In 1947, the WHO had launched the Global Influenza Surveillance Network. The Asian flu was to be its first test case, and one on which it performed extremely well. Because of the effective early warning system, public health authorities around the world were given ample notice of the pending pandemic.

One other point worth noting is that the Asian flu sparked a debate on the effectiveness of quarantine. According to the WHO, a valuable Asian flu lesson is the futility of quarantine measures which it claims: "were generally found to be ineffective, managing at best to postpone the onset of an epidemic by a few weeks to two months."[11]

Since 1957, vaccines and antibiotics have been joined by a third group of drugs—antivirals. If administered under the proper conditions, these drugs can help the body stave off flu. International organizations such as the WHO and its sister organizations, the United Nations Food and Agriculture Organization (FAO) and the World Organization for Animal Health (known by its French acronym OIE) are more aligned in terms of goals and have become more integrated in their communications. CDC and other health organizations on the national level are connected into the international system more than ever before.

Yet while the world would seem to be better prepared than it was in 1957, this is hardly the time for hubris. The technology behind vaccines has not made any significant progress in the past few decades, and the world is plagued by under-capacity in vaccine production. In addition, resistance to antibiotics is on the increase, while recent trials of antivirals call into question their usefulness in a full-blown crisis.

Hong Kong Flu: 1968-69

Of the three global flu pandemics to hit the world in the 20th century, the so-called Hong Kong flu was clearly the mildest. Earliest references to the flu appeared in the British press in July of 1968, when southeastern China was pinpointed as the source of a possible pandemic. Soon the virus turned up in Hong Kong, where due to superior medical facilities, authorities quickly identified and isolated the new strain as H3N2. By mid-August, the WHO was in a position to warn countries around the world about a possible pandemic. Most countries got off lightly with this global pandemic, but strangely not the US, where 34,000 deaths resulted from the Hong Kong flu. This particular flu pandemic had a penchant for the elderly. In contrast, in neighboring Canada, as well as across the Atlantic in the United Kingdom, the effects were less visible, in some cases, the WHO said that "deaths from influenza-like illness and pneumonia were actually lower than the year before." Even so, the Hong Kong flu pandemic is thought to have caused one million deaths around the world.[12]

False Alarm: Swine Flu of 1976

The frightening examples of the 20th century certainly provide an abundance of reasons to plan now for a future pandemic. However, another case from medical history could serve to temper resolve. The swine flu scare of 1976 is enough to make any politician, or chief executive officer for that matter, think long and hard about jumping the gun on pandemic flu.

The saga began with the death of a soldier and severe illness of several others at Fort Dix, in New Jersey. Almost immediately, there was concern that the outbreak could signal the re-emergence of a global flu pandemic along the lines of 1918.

Then-US President Gerald Ford announced an ambitious vaccination program to protect Americans against swine flu. The government spent enormous amounts of tax payers' dollars vaccinating 100 million of its citizens. But the threat never materialized. Instead, a small number of deaths occurred when some elderly people came down with Guillain Barre Syndrome, an illness where part of the body's nervous system comes under attack from the immune system.

As Mike Davis wrote in his book *The Monster at Our Door*: "From that point on, swine flu became synonymous with political fiasco."[13] And for many years to come, the topic of infectious diseases became almost taboo in the halls and corridors of Washington, DC.

The Current Wave of Flu Anxiety

While Asian media have been sporadically covering bird flu since the late 1990s, global attention to the disease really only came in 2005. Two incidents in the summer of that year served as a watershed in the development of the bird-flu story.

The first came in August, when reports began to trickle in from Central Asia and Eastern Europe of wild birds and poultry falling victim to bird flu. Suddenly the problem was no longer an Asian one. Instead, it had spread its way to the very back door of Europe, threatening not just poor Asian nations, but rich European economies such as Germany and the United Kingdom.

The second impetus came later that month when the Gulf Coast states of the US were pounded by Hurricane Katrina. The devastation and almost complete breakdown in the emergency-response system of the affected states, in particular Louisiana, shocked the world with America's inability to cope with the natural disaster. It was not long after this that avian influenza came to the fore as an important topic in domestic US politics, with President George W. Bush announcing that he would ask Congress for more than $7 billion to fund an avian flu preparedness program (the Bush administration subsequently got approval for around half that amount).

Cynics say that President Bush—embarrassed by his performance during Katrina—desperately grasped at the issue of pandemic-flu prevention as a means of showing Americans that he could protect them from natural disasters and disease just as he sought to protect them from terrorism. In reality, avian influenza and its potential to spark a flu pandemic had long been on the agenda of scientists and public-health officials in the US and many other countries. What Katrina succeeded in doing was to nudge bird flu up the Bush administration's agenda.

Bird Flu Hits Hong Kong

Whenever we speak about 1918, we have to be very careful. There is no hard evidence that can tell us definitively how the virus emerged. All we can say is that it is thought to have come about as a result of adaptive mutation of an avian virus. It is still unknown whether this took place over a prolonged period of time, or whether it happened all of a sudden.

In the case of the Asian and Hong Kong flus, we are more clear as to how they emerged. Both flu pandemics were caused by new viruses that contained both human and avian genes. This reassortment took place when a human virus and an avian virus infected the same cell at the same time, thereby making an exchange in genes possible. Where this reassortment took place is still a mystery. But up until the late 1990s at least, most scientists considered pigs as acting as a "mixing bowl" for human and avian viruses. This is because pigs' respiratory tracks provide a suitable environment where both types of viruses can thrive.

However, the outbreak of H5N1 in 1997 in Hong Kong not only presented scientists with documented proof that an avian virus—in this case H5N1—could infect humans directly, but that it could do so with fatal consequences.

In March 1997, several outbreaks of flu in poultry took place in Hong Kong, killing an estimated 7,000 chickens. At that time, scientists believed that the flu would only attack poultry, making it more of an agricultural or economic nuisance than a risk to public health. However, all that changed with the death in May of a three-year-old boy, who was later diagnosed (much later in fact, in August) as having contracted the H5N1 virus.

Even now it cannot be fully ascertained how the boy contracted the disease. But evidence points to a small pet corner in the playschool he attended that housed live chickens and ducks. It was around the same time that some of the birds died from a sudden illness that the little boy fell sick. The boy may have caught the infection through direct contact with chicken or duck feces. Yet perhaps even more curious, of 2,000 samples taken from people connected to the incident, only nine showed any signs of having come into contact with H5N1.

The case of the three-year-old boy had all the appearances of being a one-off. But in November, a second Hong Kong boy—this time a two-year old—fell ill. Again the cause was the H5N1 virus. That boy did not die. In mid-November, however, a third case emerged when a 37-year-old man was diagnosed as having H5N1-related symptoms. What followed was a continuous stream of new cases. In all, 18 people were infected. Six died. On Dec. 28, 1997, the Hong Kong government announced a cull of the territory's 1.2 million chickens. An additional half million birds of other species were destroyed. No further cases were reported after that date.

For a period of several months, imports of live chickens from mainland China were banned. New rules meant that live birds had to be segregated from one another. The measures worked. Hong Kong's terrifying brush with bird flu was over. In 2003, Hong Kong had another brief scare when a handful of nonfatal human cases were recorded. In these cases, however, it is believed the victims contracted the disease in mainland China.

Other countries have not been so fortunate. H5N1 reappeared in Southeast Asia in the winter of 2003. And by the early summer of 2006, human deaths attributed to various subtypes of H5N1 were recorded in Vietnam, Thailand, China, Cambodia, Indonesia, Azerbaijan, Iran, Iraq, Egypt and Turkey.

Sars

Hong Kong suffered another hit in 2003. This time the culprit was a hitherto unknown coronavirus—Sars. The virus is thought to have crossed the species barrier from animal to human, then evolved into a form transmissible from human to human. It first emerged in November 2002 in Guangdong Province in southern China. By March 2003, it had developed into what the WHO termed a "global threat." The disease attacked people in 26 countries, causing 774 deaths. The worst affected countries were in Asia, with China, Hong Kong, Singapore and Taiwan badly hit. The disease faded out in July 2003, but four additional cases were recorded after that.[14]

Although relatively short lived, Sars managed to inflict major damage on the economies of several Asian nations. Travel and tourism came almost to a standstill. Restaurants, bars and cinemas saw a significant drop-off in business as scared patrons elected to stay home to avoid getting infected. Many companies encouraged employees to work from home. In the space of a few short weeks, homeowners saw the value of their properties plummet and landlords were forced to slash rents. The economy faltered, and unemployment edged up.

The Sars crisis is still fresh in the minds of many Asians. It is perhaps because of this experience that awareness of the avian flu threat is high in the region. The Sars experience provides many examples of how a modern society such as Hong Kong responds to an infectious disease outbreak.

However, there is the risk that people—including business executives—conflate Sars with the threat of pandemic flu. This would be a serious mistake. As mentioned earlier, the two diseases are very different in terms of symptoms. It is arguably much easier to detect Sars. A person can carry flu for days—and infect others with it—without ever knowing he or she is a carrier. While the proportion of people killed would be lower than Sars, in terms of absolute numbers the total death toll from pandemic flu would far exceed the Sars death toll.

Even so, vital knowledge can be gained from the Sars episode. Governments and businesses can learn much about the impact of a possible pandemic on a modern society. Sars showed that peoples' behavior is rarely in correlation with the actual seriousness of the threat posed by the disease. By understanding this and crafting careful plans, it might be possible to narrow the gap between peoples' perception and the reality under a pandemic-flu scenario.

The Lessons

Hong Kong University's Malik Peiris summarized some of the scientific lessons as follows: "In 1918, a purely avian H1N1 virus seemed to have jumped species to humans. In the next pandemic in 1957, that H1N1 virus—which had by then been fully adapted to humans—re-assorted and picked up some gene segments from an avian virus. The rest of it was essentially the previous human virus, so it was a hybrid virus." The same happened in 1968. In short, the generation mechanism of the 1957-58 and 1967-68 pandemics was very different from that of 1918.

"This is relevant to the H5N1 story because it is also directly crossing to humans," said Peiris. "From here, H5N1 could directly adapt to transmission in humans, like the 1918 appears to have done, or it could re-assort with existing human virus and give rise to a hybrid virus. Both possibilities are open."

A third possibility is that the next pandemic arises from a completely different virus that has nothing to do with H5N1.

* * * * * * * * * * * * *

We must not let medical advances blind us to the fact that humanity still has not managed to rid the world of disease. In fact, just as we thought we had eradicated diseases such as tuberculosis, we find that this is far from being the case. When we become complacent, we provide disease with the opportunity to come back and infect us.

Sure, we are better prepared today when compared to 1918, historian Alfred Crosby said. "But that's like saying that building a sea wall a few feet higher will sufficiently defend us against the next tidal wave," he added.

We may have developed a vaccine that is, on the whole, effective against seasonal flu. But currently, global production capacity for producing flu vaccines is extremely limited, and the flu vaccine-preparation methods relatively antiquated when compared to drug manufacturing. While it would be unfair to lay the blame at the door of pharmaceutical companies—after all, who can blame them for not making multibillion dollar investments for something that may never happen—clearly, from a public-health perspective, it is evident that steps should be taken to urgently address these shortcomings. Thanks in part to the recent surge of interest in bird flu and pandemic flu in general, there are signs that governments and pharmaceutical companies are waking up to the gravity of the situation and are making amends.

Similar challenges are faced with regard to antiviral drugs. Questions arise as to the effectiveness of Tamiflu and other brands to fight against pandemic flu. Then there are the issues of high cost and limited supply, which has rendered them largely as drugs for the rich countries of the world.

Despite all of these limitations, we should not lose sight of the fact that we are certainly better off than those poor souls in 1918—but not by as much as we would like to think. In terms of demographics, the 1918 virus went for those in the prime of their lives. Deaths to date from the current strain of H5N1 are, quite unnervingly, also hitting a similar age group.

Quick and immediate action at the outset of a pandemic is critical. While this would seem obvious, we shouldn't expect quick and immediate response to be the norm, at least in the initial stages. Governments are notoriously reluctant to take action without concrete evidence. Yet if they wait for death tolls to mount before doing something, then it will already be too late. Emergency situations will require emergency laws. Unless the authorities are equipped with extraordinary powers—such as the ability to forcibly quarantine victims, or shut borders to international traffic—then valuable time will be lost as governments become bogged down in needless debate.

Given the importance of time, it is a little disconcerting that authorities such as the WHO say the shutting of international borders and other drastic measures will only serve to delay the onset of a pandemic by mere weeks, and will not prevent one. Yet even a breathing space of one or two weeks could make a huge difference in terms of preparing the medical authorities for the impending crisis, or give scientists extra leeway for isolating the virus and working on possible vaccine development.

Geography plays a critical role. In 1918, not all places were hit at the same time or with the same intensity. The city of Brest, in France, was the gateway to Europe for thousands of American soldiers during the war. Similarly, modern-day crossroads of the world—cities such as London, New York, Hong Kong, Singapore and Dubai—are particularly vulnerable to becoming epicenters of pandemic flu.

Other lessons that can be gleaned are more practical if somewhat morbid. One of the biggest problems of 1918 was a complete breakdown in the process of collecting and burying dead bodies. As the pandemic spiked, hospitals were inundated with patients to the extent that they could not cope. The number of trained nurses was so low that local governments had to appeal to the able-bodied to volunteer. Not surprisingly, few did. These insights remind us that, no matter how detailed our preparedness plan might be, our basic infrastructure needs to be adequate enough to deal with the enormous strain that would be placed on it should a flu pandemic the likes of 1918 occur. While there is no hard data to substantiate the effectiveness of minimizing public gatherings, anecdotal evidence from 1918 suggests that it would be the prudent thing to do; the benefits (mainly psychological) of using face masks; and the very real benefits of enhanced hygiene practices, such as hand washing.

Leaving these practical points aside, past pandemics provide a very interesting window into human nature as it transforms under pandemic conditions. And it is not a pretty sight. Howard Markel of the University of Michigan describes in his book *When Germs Travel* how xenophobia and discrimination are quick to appear as soon as a pandemic or epidemic occurs. Describing an outbreak of bubonic plague in San Francisco's Chinatown in 1900, Markel describes the "all-too-reflexive impulse Americans often have in establishing quarantine or public-health policy based on race, ethnicity, or social disenfranchisement."[15]

Another critical consideration is communication. In 1918, global mass communications as we know it today simply did not exist. In addition, as historian Alfred Crosby pointed out, the daily lives of many citizens in many countries, including the US and the United Kingdom, were thrown into chaos because of the ongoing war; many people were either too preoccupied with other matters or simply too weary to take much notice of the influenza that was sweeping the world.[16] Today, that situation is very different, as news organizations report the daily minutiae of disease developments from around the world. "Thanks to mass media, this time we would get mass panic," predicted Crosby.

It is reassuring to note that the later pandemics of the 1950s and 1960s had considerably less of an impact on global and national economies than Spanish flu. The same cannot be said about Sars which had a huge, albeit short-term impact, on the economies of several countries, mainly in Asia. Given that Sars occurred in recent memory, in a business environment largely unchanged from that of today's, it is not surprising then that it provides some of the most important lessons for business executives considering ways to prepare for a flu pandemic.

Endnotes

1   *The History of the Peloponnesian War*, by Thucydides & Translated by Richard Crawley, see: http://classics.mit.edu/Thucydides/pelopwar.html

2   *World Epidemics: A Cultural Chronology of Disease from Prehistory to the Era of Sars*, Mary Ellen Snodgrass, McFarland & Company (2003)

3   *Epidemics and History: Disease, Power and Imperialism*, Sheldon Watts, Yale University Press (1999) page 167

4   *America's Forgotten Pandemic: The Influenza of 1918*, Alfred W. Crosby, Cambridge University Press (2003)

5   *Flu: The Story of the Great Influenza Pandemic of 1918 and the Search for the Virus That Caused It*, Gina Kolata FSG (1999), page 12

6   *The Great Influenza: The Epic Story of the Deadliest Plague in History*, John M. Barry, Penguin (2004), page 453

7   *World Epidemics: A Cultural Chronology of Disease from Prehistory to the Era of Sars*, Mary Ellen Snodgrass, McFarland & Company (2003), page 280

8   WHO Handbook for Journalists: Influenza Pandemic, WHO, December 2005, page 5

9   "Avian influenza: assessing the pandemic threat," *WHO*, January 2005, page 29

10 Ibid. page 29

11 Ibid. page 29

12 Ibid. page 31

13 *The Monster at Our Door*, Mike Davis, The New Press (2005), page 43

14 "WHO guidelines for the global surveillance of severe acute respiratory syndrome (Sars)." Updated recommendations October 2004, page 6

15 *When Germs Travel: Six Major Epidemics That Have Invaded America Since 1900 and the Fears They Have Unleashed*; Howard Markel; Pantheon (2004), page 74

16 *America's Forgotten Pandemic: The Influenza of 1918*, Alfred W. Crosby, Cambridge University Press (2003), page 18

Chapter Three

Lessons from the Future?

"[T]he power of mathematical modeling is
that you can foretell 10 years in advance what
might happen."

Gabriel Leung
University of Hong Kong's School of Public Health

History provides valuable lessons for pandemic planning. But what if we could predict the future? Not surprisingly, there is no crystal ball, no supercomputer that when fed with copious amounts of data and statistics will churn out the answer to the question on many minds: When will the next pandemic flu strike?

Yet while it is impossible to predict the timing, it is possible to build predictive models that can help us better prepare for future events. Around the world, a small, but growing number of mathematicians, scientists and economists are striving to increase our ability to predict what a future pandemic will look like and to help authorities and businesses to plan for it more effectively.

This chapter outlines some of the advancements in pandemic modeling in the world of science. Subsequent chapters will take a closer look at the insights that can be gleaned from macro- and microeconomic models.

In the early 1990s, few could predict the massive impact HIV/AIDS would have on the world. Few, except Professor Roy Anderson of Oxford University. Anderson carefully studied the disease among sex workers in Kenya. Then, using a model that drew more from the laws of physics than biology, he plotted a graph that "predicted" how the killer disease would explode in the future.[1] This was in direct contradiction to other studies of that period which suggested that HIV/AIDS would disappear from the planet within a few years.[2] Over time, Anderson's approach was shown to be correct as the real data that emerged over the subsequent 10-year period was almost identical to his original predictions. Anderson's study was to prove to be an enormous breakthrough. His predictive curve foretold the nightmare that was in store for global health and gave an advance warning to the world's health authorities of the sheer enormity of the task that lay ahead.

To be sure, not all mathematical models are so successful at predicting the future. And influenza is a particularly difficult disease to model because of the enormous number of variables that would need to be taken into account. Yet even the simplest of models can help governments and businesses prepare for a pandemic and edge public-health and corporate planning closer to fact and away from fiction.

Most of the pandemic-flu related models that are currently doing the rounds have been built with the needs of policymakers in mind. But they can still be useful for business executives charged with pandemic planning. At the very least, by studying some of these models and becoming familiar with their underlying concepts, executives can build fluency in the language of influenza. They will become savvier about the factors at play in a pandemic, and this understanding should help them to develop better business continuity plans and make better decisions in the event of a flu pandemic.

What Can Models Do?

Models can make the abstract concept of a pandemic flu outbreak more real and thereby facilitate planning. Even elementary models can help us get a sense of scale and impact of flu pandemic in terms of number of infected, number of deaths, number requiring hospitalization, etc.

FluAid, developed by the CDC in the US, is one example. Although still officially in its test phase, the software is designed to help public-health officials gauge the impact a flu pandemic might have on their communities. (The software is freely available online at http://www2.cdc.gov/od/fluaid/default.htm.) Users were asked to key in data such as estimated mortality rates for three different scenarios ("minimum," "most likely" and "maximum"). The program then calculated the likely impact in terms of the number of people that will seek hospitalization, the expected number of outpatients, as well as the total number of deaths under the three scenarios' terms. But the model doesn't tell health workers how the disease will evolve, where people will become sick. Health officials outside the US have also used FluAid to estimate the impact on their healthcare systems. Using data from past pandemics, Singapore's Ministry of Health estimated that 450,000 of Singapore's 4.6 million inhabitants could develop a "mild form of the disease." This would result in the hospitalization of 11,000 residents and the death of 1,900 people in the city state.[3]

FluAid could easily be modified by corporations and used in scenario building for a flu pandemic. By developing a calculator that looks at total number of employees, their demographics, location, and other parameters, and assigning different employees different risk factors, under various scenarios (a high, medium, or low attack rate; a high, medium, or low mortality) companies can get a better feel for the impact a pandemic might have on their employees. This approach is more nuanced than predicting flu-related absenteeism using a flat rate of, say, 30%. Similarly, models also could be developed by companies to estimate the impact on suppliers or markets.

Tools such as FluAid, however, offer little advice on how best to *handle* a pandemic outbreak. One model developed by Neil Ferguson, mathematical biologist at the Imperial College London, aims to provide public-health officials with somewhat more practical guidance.[4] Using a computer model that mapped the evolution of a hypothetical bird flu outbreak in rural Thailand, researchers showed that, under certain conditions, it might be possible to stop human-to-human transmission of bird flu in its tracks at an early stage, and deny the virus the chance to escalate into a global pandemic. In the midst of so much bird flu doom and gloom, the study offered encouragement that the world is not totally helpless in the face of an avian flu-triggered pandemic. The findings suggested that with proper well-informed strategies, it could be possible to win the war on H5N1.

Whether the assumptions of some of this model can be mirrored in real life remains to be seen. First, there needs to be a sufficient supply of antiviral drugs that are effective against the strain of flu that is threatening to explode into a pandemic. But even this basic assumption is questionable. There is some doubt about the effectiveness of antivirals such as Tamiflu (oseltamivir) or Relenza (zanamivir). It cannot be said for sure that they will work. And even if they did work, would there be enough to ship to the scene of an outbreak? How easy would it be to ship Tamiflu from warehouses in

Switzerland or even Singapore, and rapidly distribute them to remote corners of countries such as Thailand or Laos?

These considerations aside, the research suggested that geographically targeted prophylaxis of antivirals together with social distancing measures—closures of schools, offices, factories, etc.—could prevent a flu epidemic from becoming a pandemic. If the virus were not stopped in its tracks, it would only be a matter of weeks, if not days, before it spread to Bangkok, from where its international debut would only be a short plane ride away.

In a subsequent study, Ferguson and colleagues expanded the scope of their research to examine strategies for reducing the impact of an influenza pandemic by examining the cases of the US and the United Kingdom.[5] The main findings suggested by this mathematical model included:

- *Border restrictions*: Closing the frontiers to international traffic will not stop pandemic flu from entering a country. At best, such measures can only serve to delay the onslaught of the virus. The model suggested that border restrictions together with internal travel restrictions could only allow governments to buy between two and three weeks of "extra" time.

- *School closures*: Closing schools during the peak of a pandemic could help reduce peak attack rates by as much as 40%, the researchers found. However, they hastened to add that such closures will have very little real long-term impact on overall attack rates of the pandemic. Instead, the model suggested that the isolation of flu victims as well as quarantining entire households could be more effective.

- *Vaccine stockpiling:* The model suggested that advanced stockpiling of a vaccine could have a "substantial impact on attack rates, even if its efficacy was less than a vaccine matched against the pandemic strain."

Ferguson and his colleagues are by no means the only mathematicians and scientists that are exploring influenza pandemic strategies by building mathematical models. Other notable leaders in the field include Ira Longini—professor in the Department of Biostatistics, School of Public Health and Community Medicine at the University of Washington—and Timothy Germann at the Los Alamos National Laboratory.[6]

All of these mathematicians face the same reality: modeling for a pandemic is fraught with challenges. The number of different parameters that are required to build a realistic model is staggering, and the dynamics of a pandemic much more erratic than traditional risk modeling techniques can accommodate.

Even so, studies such as those by Ferguson have implications for business. The findings underline an important point in pandemic flu preparedness: speed—or rather the lack of it—kills. The private sector should lend its full support, in whatever way it can, to assist public-health authorities' attempts to rapidly quash the virus at source. This could mean providing logistical support to get antivirals to the right location as speedily as possible. Or it could mean generally being responsive to a government's social distancing requests.

These, and other studies[7] also serve to drive home the point that, even in the face of a looming pandemic, there are actions which can be taken that could defuse the threat or at least minimize its impact. The message that governments and businesses are not totally helpless against a flu pandemic is perhaps the most valuable lesson of all.

Human Behavior and Pandemics

Gabriel Leung and colleagues at the Hong Kong University's School of Public Health are developing a model aimed at examining how people's psychological response during a pandemic influences how a virus is spread. Using a detailed series of psychobehavioral surveillance data obtained during the Sars crisis, the researchers measure how people's psychological state correlate with their willingness to take measures to protect themselves from the contagious disease, such as whether they chose to wear a face mask, or to refrain from visiting public places such as restaurants and cinemas. Clearly, willingness to adapt these types of behavior is crucial to curbing the spread of the disease, since doing so reduces direct contact between people. This, in turn, minimizes the number of people an infected person could transmit the disease to.

Leung said that at the peak of the Sars outbreak, people who were "slightly anxious," were most likely to take personal protective measures. Not surprisingly, those who were not concerned at all ignored calls from public-health officials to take precautionary measures. But perhaps the most noteworthy finding is that people who described themselves as "very anxious" also opted not to take health officials' advice. It is as if their fear had paralyzed them from taking action.

By the time the end of the pandemic was in sight, however, a very different picture had emerged, and more people were taking protective measures. Leung attributes this change in people's psychological state primarily to the influence of the media.

This understanding of the pivotal role the media can play in influencing behavior has led Leung and fellow University of Hong Kong academic, Thomas Abraham, director of the university's Public Health Media Project, to conduct further analyses of Sars-era data. Their hope is that in the event of a pandemic, they will be able to help the Hong Kong authorities craft media messages that will be effective in shaping public perceptions of the outbreak and positively influence people's behavior.

"Hong Kong is in a very fortunate position because Sars has provided researchers with a gold mine of data to study the behavior of citizens under a pandemic situation," explained Leung. "We have travel data on a daily basis, we have restaurant receipts, [etc.] We can see how a population responds in a media savvy age."

By studying the public's reactions to the various ways the health authorities intervened to stem the Sars crisis—including the use of quarantine, isolation, antiviral and contact tracing—the Hong Kong University team hopes to evaluate the relative effectiveness of the different methods from a human behavior perspective. This would allow governments and companies to spend time and money on those activities that yield greater results.

For business executives, the main message of this research is the power of communication. A good communications strategy can allay fears. An ineffective one could serve only to spread panic. Managers should never lose sight of human behavior in a pandemic situation. It is the wild card that can make or break even the best laid plans.

Looking to the Future

Given the billions of dollars that international organizations, governments and corporations are setting aside to prepare for a flu pandemic, there has been comparatively little investment in terms of resources and money devoted to pandemic-flu modeling. Hopefully, that may change in the near future as governments and corporations begin to better grasp the potential benefits of models for guiding planning.

Steven Riley, assistant professor at the University of Hong Kong's Department of Community Medicine, foresaw a change in the type of modeling that will be conducted. Up to now, models have tended to measure the impact of a pandemic (FluAid), or have tried to identify ways to stamp out an outbreak before it becomes a full-fledged pandemic (the Ferguson study).

"There is a lot of talk about how to identify outbreaks, or potentially how to control one," said Riley. "But there is not a lot of detailed thinking about exactly what is best to do once pandemic flu begins to spread." We should expect to see more modeling focused on devising what he terms "mitigation strategies."

"Mitigation indicates that you don't expect to stop a pandemic completely," said Riley. "You expect to reduce the impact of [the pandemic], but it will progress through a large proportion of the population."

This shift in the nature of pandemic modeling will raise a whole series of new questions, said Riley. For example, whereas studies to date have evaluated traditional intervention techniques such as the effectiveness of quarantine, isolation, antiviral drugs and social distancing, the trend is toward expanding the scope of modeling to help answer such questions as *when* and *how* to best use antiviral drugs.

But first, Riley believed public-health goals will need to be defined more specifically. For example, in the event of a flu pandemic, is the aim to reduce the total number of deaths? Or is it to minimize the number of deaths among key workers? Or is the goal to reduce the duration of the pandemic for citizens?

"There are a lot of difficult questions that are not being answered, or even really being asked in a particularly formal way at the moment," said Riley.

Endnotes

1   Anderson et al., The Spread of HIV-1 in Africa: Sexual Contact and the Predicted Demograhic Impact of AIDS. *Nature*, Aug. 15, 1991, page 581-589

2   Bregman and Langmuir, "Farr's Law Applied to AIDS Projections." *Journal of the American Medical Association*, Mar. 16, 1990, page 1522-1525

3   "A bird flu pandemic could kill 1,900 in Singapore," by Elaine Young, *Straits Times*, Dec. 10, 2005

4   "Strategies for containing an emerging influenza pandemic in Southeast Asia," *Nature*, Vol. 437/8 September 2005

5   "Strategies for mitigating an influenza pandemic," Neil M. Fergusson et al., Nature, April 26, 2006

6   http://www.lanl.gov/news/index.php?fuseaction=home.story&story_id=8171

7   See http://www.bio-itworld.com/newsitems/2005/dec2005/12-05-05-news-avian-flu; and http://www.nigms.nih.gov/Initiatives/MIDAS/

Chapter Four

The Economic Impact of Pandemic Flu

"If all economists were laid end to end,
they would not reach a conclusion."

— George Bernard Shaw

W hen economists told Senator Bill Frist that a severe flu pandemic could cause a 5% reduction in US GDP, the senate majority leader from Tennessee wasn't fazed: "A \$675 billion hit to the economy is, without question, a grim prognosis," Frist told reporters in December 2005, but quickly added: "[But] our hands are not tied." Frist believes that, if the proper steps are taken now in advance of a pandemic, America can drastically reduce the potential damage to its economy.[1]

During his two-decade long medical career, 54-year-old Frist performed more than 150 heart and lung transplants. As a politician, he was a leading advocate for increased global funding for HIV/AIDS, and a volunteer in post-tsunami Sri Lanka. He also witnessed firsthand the chaotic aftermath of Hurricane Katrina in New Orleans in August 2005.

In late 2005, unhappy with the level of economic analysis that was available on pandemic flu, Frist asked the US Congressional Budgetary Office (CBO) to step in. The CBO is the main congressional agency charged with reviewing congressional budgets and other legislative initiatives that have an impact on the US government's budget. Every year its 235 employees prepare some 2,000 budget estimations of legislation being considered by Congress, and several dozen analytical reports.

In response to Frist's request, the CBO produced an assessment[2] of the macroeconomic impacts of pandemic influenza on the US economy. Its report was perhaps the most comprehensive analysis of pandemic flu on an economy up to that point. The results of the analysis were startling.

Economics of Pandemic Flu

In the past, when economists calculated the cost of a disease, they tended to focus on a rather narrow data set. They wanted to know how many people died prematurely as a result of the disease, how their deaths affected productivity and how their lost future incomes affected supply. These are known as direct costs.

In more recent years, economists have begun to take a broader approach in calculating the real cost of disease. This includes factoring in indirect costs arising from fear, panic, confusion and other psychological factors.

These psychological factors can be controlled, said Frist. This can be done by having a plan, and communicating that plan clearly to the public.

"Failing to effectively communicate with the public—both before and during the pandemic—is analogous with having a fire escape plan for your home but neglecting to share the plan with your family," he said. When a fire breaks out, family members will end up jumping out the window even though there is a ladder under the bed, the senator warned.

Economists would describe the factors at play in a pandemic-struck society in a slightly different way. They prefer to talk about "shocks" to the economy from the supply side and from the demand side.

Supply side inputs include labor, logistics, and health and medical care. In the CBO study, the impact of a flu pandemic on labor supply in the US scenario is enormous. One million Americans are forced to stop working either because they are too ill, too afraid to turn up to work, too preoccupied with caring for sick relatives, or simply have died from the disease. CBO estimates that, regardless of whether the pandemic is mild or severe, 30% of the population could miss up to three weeks of work. In the severe scenario, of 90 million infected Americans, two million could die.

But that's not all. Supply chains would be severely disrupted as transportation, especially across borders, comes to a standstill. The supply of medical services and medication would, to say the very least, be severely curtailed, with both flu and nonflu patients being unable to access proper care. All told, these supply side costs would account for a 3% drop in US GDP.

Of a total 5% slide in GDP, the remaining two percentage points would come from demand side effects, the CBO economists predict. Demand inputs include consumer, corporate and government spending. With consumers forced or choosing to shut themselves away from the pandemic, the travel, restaurant and entertainment industries could experience drops in demand of up to 80%. Retail sales could plummet by as much as 25%. To be sure, demand for healthcare and related products would surge.

In dollar terms the 5% GDP drop would amount to $675 billion, constituting a particularly nasty economic downturn and worse than most of the past recessions which, according to the CBO, averaged drops of around 4.7%.

Of course, those supply- and demand-shock numbers are for the severe scenario. In this version, about one in three Americans contract the flu, and the proportion of sick people that die is also high (2.5% of all infected die). Infection patterns under these scenarios mirror closely the Spanish flu of 1918.

But even under the mild scenario—more akin to the Asian flu of 1957-58 or the Hong Kong flu of 1968-69—the CBO predicts that supply side effects would result in a 1% reduction in GDP, while demand side effects would knock another 0.5% off. In this scenario, the infection rate is slightly lower (25%) but the mortality rate at 1.14% is still alarming. In the case of the US, this would translate to 75 million infections, resulting in 100,000 fatalities. This is still three times the number of people that die annually in the US from seasonal flu.

Overblown or Understated?

The CBO could be greatly overstating the potential economic impact of pandemic flu. After all, it's next to impossible to pinpoint to the last dollar the damage a flu pandemic might cause. However, its basic approach—separating the causes of an economic downturn into direct and indirect effects—has been validated by evidence from the Sars outbreak.

By the time the threat from Sars finally subsided, it had hit 29 countries on three continents, resulting in more than 8,000 cases of infection and a total of 774 deaths. Asian economies bore the brunt of the disease, both in terms of mortality and negative economic impact, with China, Hong Kong, Taiwan and Singapore among the worst affected.

But Toronto was also hard hit. Canadian economist Sherry Cooper describes the disproportionate economic impact the disease had on the city of Toronto compared to the actual health threat. In the period between March and June 2003, there were 252 cases reported in Toronto, resulting in the deaths of 44 people.

Around 15,000 people had to be quarantined. Some hospitals reached surge capacity and nonessential surgery had to be greatly curtailed or postponed. Many schools were closed. Foreigners refused to travel to the city and the WHO advised against doing so, Cooper told a February 2006 seminar on business pandemic planning in Minneapolis.

Many other cities and countries made it clear that visitors from Toronto were not welcome. Conferences were canceled. People shunned restaurants and public places, with some people who associated Sars with Asians even boycotting Chinese restaurants out of fear, Cooper explained. The city's tourism and hospitality industry was crushed. Air Canada—long plagued with financial difficulties— declared bankruptcy. What followed was an unprecedented economic downturn in the city whose reach extended far beyond the province of Ontario to affect the entire country. Cooper said it took Canada two years to fully recover from the impact of Sars which saw GDP growth fall from 3% in the first quarter of 2003 to 1.2% in the second quarter.

Most of the economic contraction in Canada came from the "direct" costs that Frist mentioned. A drop in demand for travel, tourism, arts and entertainment, hospitality and retail services— largely spurred by people's often irrational response to the disease— was the main reason for the economic nosedive. There is little evidence of any significant impact on supply-side factors.

A similar pattern emerged in Asia, where Sars wreaked even greater havoc on Hong Kong. One estimate puts GDP falling by 2% in the region during the second quarter of 2003. In their study of the economic impact of Sars, Professors Alan Siu and Richard Wong, economists at the University of Hong Kong, measured the impact of Sars on different segments of the economy. They noted that retail sales figures in March 2003 were HK$14.17 billion ($1.8 billion), down 6.1% from the same period a year earlier. Airlines fared even worse, with passenger traffic down by as much as 77% in April 2003 from the same month the year before. According to figures from the Hong Kong Tourism Board, 15.5 million visitors came to Hong Kong during 2003, down 6.2% on the previous year—a reduction largely attributed to Sars. About a quarter of Hong Kong residents canceled their overseas trips, perhaps sensing they might be unwelcome visitors in certain countries.[3]

Yet this study also showed that, as in Canada, Sars had little supply-side impact in Hong Kong. The territory's export activities were not affected, and there was no apparent reduction in cross-border traffic figures during the period March to September of 2003. Similarly, there were no major disruptions to Hong Kong-owned factories across the border in the mainland China province of Guangdong.

Yet most estimates of the economic impact of the Sars crisis do not tell the full story. Many such estimates are merely snapshots of individual economies at a specific time, and so greatly underestimate the true cost of the outbreak. South Korean economist Jong-Wha Lee and Australian economist Warwick McKibbin developed a model in 2003 that attempted to conduct a comprehensive analysis of the impact of Sars by factoring in the linkages that exist between different sectors of the economy and between one economy and another.[4] The two economists set out to estimate the global cost of Sars by examining its effect on consumption, and probing investment behavior that arose from the cost and risk of doing business. They factored in the interdependencies among economies and the role of investor confidence. Using this approach, their estimates of the cost of Sars, $40 billion, suggest that even a short-lived epidemic packed a mighty economic punch. This ground-breaking study by Lee and McKibbin was to serve as the basis for a more recent model developed by McKibbin—this time with colleague Alexandra Sidorenko—that measures just how much an influenza pandemic would cost the global economy.

Economic Impact of Pandemic Influenza

The picture painted by the CBO for the United States economy is grim. Taken from a global economic perspective, the view is even worse.

"I hate doing 'the world is going to end' type of scenarios," said McKibbin. But that is precisely what he and Sidorenko of the Australian National University did in February 2006.[5] The pair studied the global impact of a pandemic flu— and the results weren't pretty: more than 140 million people dead, and global GDP slashed by $4.4 trillion, or 12.6%. Their estimates make those by the World Bank or the Asian Development Bank look almost reassuring.

In November 2005, Milan Brahmbhatt, lead economist with the World Bank's East Asia and Pacific region, told a bird-flu conference in Geneva that the global impact could top $800 billion, or roughly 2% of the world's global GDP. In order to arrive at this global estimate, World Bank economists relied heavily on the experience from Sars, but Brahmbhatt conceded that: "It is fair to assume the immediate shock during a bird-flu epidemic could be even larger and last longer than Sars."[6]

The ADB agreed with this assessment and said:

"These [economic impact] estimates suggest that avian flu would lead to a severe economic shock in the Asia and Pacific region, with economic consequences in the range of $100 billion–$300 billion. At its worst, this would essentially halt economic growth for one year and throw the world into an economic recession, the first global recession since 1982."[7]

In their report, *Global Macroeconomic Consequences of Pandemic Influenza*, McKibbin and Sidorenko go beyond any of the other analyses in terms of the sophistication of the assumptions. Even the

CBO report, while excellent, focuses only on domestic US considerations. But what makes the current threat more frightening than past pandemics is the globalized state of the world economy. Globalization has brought a level of interconnectivity and interdependence between countries and economies never seen before, which could serve to even further magnify the negative economic effects of pandemic flu.

These global linkages and interdependencies—including both financial and trading ties—have been factored into the Australians' model. The duo describes four different pandemic scenarios: mild, moderate, severe and ultra. The first two scenarios roughly correspond to the virulence of the Hong Kong and Asian flus. The last two scenarios use fatality rates from the Spanish flu, with the "ultra" pandemic using a rate from the higher end of the range. In all scenarios, the attack rate is 30%.

Once again, the message is clear: Even a mild flu outbreak could result in 1.4 million dead and major economic losses to the global economy, with one percentage point—or a staggering $330 billion— knocked off of global GDP.

If this is the mild scenario, what then do the economists foresee under the "ultra" case? They estimate that 142 million people would lose their lives, some economies would contract by as much as 50% and global GDP could drop by 12.6%, or $4.4 trillion.

Not all countries would be affected equally. For example, McKibbin and Sidorenko anticipated a flow of capital from the affected economies to the less affected countries. Their model shows that equity markets would fall while bond markets would rally. With equities, the fall is not as much as expected, especially when examined over a one-year period. This, McKibbin explained, is because after the initial shock to equity prices, markets soon reassume a long-term perspective, looking to the future where they see an eventual recovery in demand.

Central banks will face a dilemma under a pandemic scenario. On the one hand, a drop in demand will result in deflation as people stop buying goods. On the other hand, supply-side costs will increase, resulting in inflationary pressure. How governments respond to this will have significant consequences for economies. The trade-off between tightening and loosening monetary policy, McKibbin said, will be similar to the choices many Asian governments had to face during the Asian financial crisis of 1997. Countries that have currencies that are pegged to other currencies will be especially hard-hit, irrespective of where a pandemic may first appear. Whether it originates in Asia or elsewhere, markets where the local currency is pegged to the dollar could be in for a rocky ride, the authors say.

Developing countries would be affected more than the developed countries, the duo say, because they experience a greater "mortality shock" due to their lack of infrastructure and poor health systems. This will be compounded by sinking trade volumes and the flight of investors, who will rush to pull funds from these countries.

Not Everyone is Convinced

Not all economists believe such bleak scenarios will come to pass. Rob Subbaraman, Lehman Brothers' senior economist for Asia, said the bank's "inclination is *not* to view the future as all gloom and doom."[8] An important factor underlying Subbaraman's upbeat take is Sars:

> *"Compared to the last three flu pandemics, Sars scarcely registered on the calamity scale. One reason is that the Sars virus was relatively mild. But a more crucial reason, we believe, is that the world in 2003 was much better prepared to cope."*

Subbaraman went on to say that an avian flu outbreak is more likely to be a regional *epidemic* rather than a global *pandemic*. Three scenarios are foreseen by the Hong Kong-based analyst:

In the first scenario, an outbreak is confined to the poultry sector. According to the report, the poultry sector accounts for 2% of the Asia's GDP. A drop of 20% in demand would result in a loss of 0.4 percentage points off regional GDP.

In the second scenario, the flu epidemic spreads to the travel and tourism industry and other service sectors. The net impact is 1.5 percentage points to two percentage points off of GDP in the quarters where the outbreak peaks.

There is a low probability that the final scenario would occur. In this case, the virus is more virulent and has a longer life. For a pandemic like this, Subbaraman said that the "economic impact could be much larger, with the recovery taking much longer" than was the case with Sars. Despite his comparatively upbeat take on the economic impact of a flu pandemic, Lehman Brothers listed avian influenza as one of their top 10 risks for the Asian economy in 2006.

Conclusions

Economists may disagree on precisely how much pandemic flu could cost the world economy, but most agree that, even if the next influenza pandemic turns out to be mild, it will still have a major impact on the world economy.

The main reason for this of course is human behavior. People react to threats in many different ways and it seems probable that an outbreak of pandemic influenza—no matter how mild—will be greeted with fear and panic. It is these psychological factors that can be the real source of damage to an economy as people withdraw from society and demand drops, setting in motion a downward economic spiral.

But the message from people like Frist is equally clear. Even though it might be impossible to eradicate fear from every man, woman and child around the world, by taking action now, these psychological fears can be reduced. If companies, community groups, organizations and governments take the initiative—ahead of the emergence of a flu pandemic—there is a good chance that people could be sufficiently educated on the true extent of the threats posed by pandemic influenza.

In this respect, companies are well-placed to begin the process of allaying fears by developing logical business continuity plans that are communicated effectively within the organization and to related parties such as suppliers. And, as Chapter 5 shows, some companies are already well on the way to developing and implementing such plans to deal with pandemic influenza.

Endnotes

1   See http://frist.senate.gov/index.cfm?FuseAction=Speeches.Detail&Speech_id=322
2   "A Potential Influenza Pandemic: Possible Macroeconomic Effects and Policy Issues," The Congress of the United States Congressional Budget Office, Dec. 8, 2005
3   "Economic Impact of Sars: The Case of Hong Kong," Alan Siu, Y.C. Richard Wong, *Asian Economic Papers*, August 2004, Vol. 3, No. 1, Pages 62-83
4   "Globalization and Disease: The Case of Sars," Jong-Wha Lee and Warwick J. McKibbin, Brookings Discussion Papers in *International Economics*, July 2003 (Revised).
5   "Global Macroeconomic Consequences of Pandemic Influenza," Warwick J. McKibbin and Alexandra Sidorenko, Lowy Institute for International Policy, February 2006
6   "Avian Flu: Economic Losses Could Top $800 Billion," *The World Bank Group*, Nov. 8, 2005
7   Asian Development Outlook 2006, ADB, page 26
8   Rob Subbaraman and Wenzhong Fan in *Asia Ex-Japan Weekly Economic Monitor*, Lehman Brothers, Nov. 11, 2005

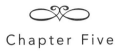

Chapter Five

The Impact on Industry

"The business community can no longer
afford to play a minor role in planning the
response to a pandemic. For the world to
have critical goods and services during a
pandemic, industry heads must stockpile raw
materials for production and preplan
distribution and transportation support."

Dr. Michael T. Osterholm[1]
Director, Center for Infectious Disease Research and
Policy, *University of Minnesota*

Imagine the following scenario. An airline passenger on a flight
from Hong Kong to London develops flu-like symptoms,
rousing the attention of his fellow passengers. Soon, the airline
crew has scrambled to take action, notifying airport authorities in
London that someone on board the flight may have bird flu.
Wanting to be on the safe side, the panicked British airport
authorities quarantine the entire aircraft. But after isolating
passengers for several days, the incident turns out to be a false alarm.
The passenger had a normal seasonal flu, and no trace of H5N1
is found.

Guess who gets stuck with the bill for the entire ordeal? The
airline company, of course.

For Andrew Herdman, director general of the Association of Asia Pacific Airlines, based in Kuala Lumpur, Malaysia, the above scenario is one of his biggest concerns. He worries that the real threat to his association's members is not so much bird flu itself, but rather, hasty decisions made in reaction to an uncertain flu threat.

Such fear could translate into a massive drop in demand for air travel, an industry notoriously sensitive to wars, terrorism and other shocks. The stakes are high: last year the industry raked in global revenues of $400 billion, but generated more than $3 trillion in economic activity overall—8% of the world's GNP. It employs a staggering 29 million people worldwide.[2] And if an H5N1 or a pandemic flu crisis cripples the airline industry, the effects would spread rapidly through the entire global economy.

Herdman knows just how vulnerable the airline industry is. He has more than two decades of experience in the business, including a stint as director of corporate affairs with responsibility for crisis management at Swire Pacific, parent company of the Hong Kong-based airline Cathay Pacific. In the past 10 years, he has witnessed enormous swings in demand triggered by the Asian financial crisis of 1997, the fallout from the terror attacks of Sept. 11, 2001, the Sars crisis of 2003, and, most recently, the Boxing Day tsunami of 2004. Perhaps because of this long experience with such disasters, Herdman is coolheaded about the possibility of a bird flu pandemic.

"Avian flu is way down the list of would-be health threats to people in their ordinary lives," he said. Diseases such as malaria or dengue fever pose greater threats to traveler safety, said Herdman. But facts like this will surely get lost in the confusion in the event of a bird-flu epidemic (or an influenza pandemic). As governments and international organizations speed up their efforts to fight bird flu, the airline industry could likely suffer from the panicked, ill-advised decisions of others.

It's tempting to say: "'Stop the world!' and shut down international travel," said Herdman. Such dramatic moves are appealing to politicians who feel compelled to take high-profile action—any action—in the face of an uncertain threat. "It's a 'protect my citizens, keep out those foreigners with those foreign diseases' kind of attitude," he said.

Herdman said that travel restrictions introduced during the Sars crisis serve as a powerful example of what *not* to do in a pandemic. At the height of the crisis, some countries imposed severe travel restrictions. Malaysia at one point stopped issuing tourist visas to would-be visitors from China and Hong Kong. "Many of those restrictions didn't pass the test of rationality," said Herdman.

Herdman said that while we don't know how effective travel restrictions and other measures might be, one thing we do know for sure is how disruptive such methods can be to the economy and society, and the "massive" costs associated with such a move. Herdman estimated a ballpark figure for the economic impact of Sars on the airline industry at "several billion dollars," a figure consistent with estimates from the Asian Development Bank of a $30 billion loss to the economy in Asia alone.[3]

The Sars episode raises other reasons to question the usefulness of travel restrictions under a pandemic flu. Sars had certain telltale symptoms, such as high body temperature, which made it easier to pinpoint sick passengers during screening at airports. That's not the case with flu, since carriers of the virus may show no symptoms, at least in the early stages of infection. Even if some effective screening test were found, airports could be thrown into chaos just trying to administer it. Apart from banning international travel altogether, it would be impossible to effectively restrict the travel of all flu victims.

Sars was also a relatively short-lived crisis, lasting around half a year. Pandemic flu can come in waves over a period of one or two years. Intense screening of passengers for such a prolonged period would not just be logistically challenging, it would also be incredibly expensive.

Herdman was convinced that the main challenge to the airline industry will be dealing with an inevitable fall-off in demand. Yet even on this front, the options open to airline executives are limited. By expanding its use of operating leases, an airline could hypothetically increase its fleet's flexibility, since the carrier has the right to return the aircraft to the leasing company should demand suddenly fall. "The difficulty is that flexibility comes at a price," explained Herdman. "You've got to weigh up if you want the flexibility. It's the old rent or buy dilemma."

But Herdman said the airline industry is beginning to embrace the concept of business continuity planning. For now, airlines are focusing on basic steps, such as educating crew about how to handle suspected cases among passengers. The only problem with this approach is that one in three airline staff could be out sick, or tending to sick relatives.

Different Industries, Different Impact

Beyond airlines, how would other industries fare under a pandemic flu scenario? It's impossible to predict exactly how a pandemic would play out in different sectors of the global economy. But the US CBO analysis provides as good a starting point as any.[4]

Loosely basing its estimations on Sars, the CBO first considered whether an industry had a high degree of social interaction. Do people have to come into direct contact with other human beings in order to consume the products or services on offer from a given industry? Not surprisingly, industries that involve greater social interaction saw the highest drop-off in demand. Table 3 summarizes the different drops in demand for various sectors of the economy under two scenarios: severe and mild.

As might be expected, the airline industry, as well as other transport-related sectors such as rail and logistics, would be the hardest hit. The CBO foresaw these sectors experiencing a 67% drop-off in demand under a severe scenario, and a 17% decline under a mild scenario. Even so, transportation is not the worst affected sector. That dubious honor goes to service providers in the arts and entertainment sector, such as movie theaters, as well as hotels, tour operators and restaurants (demand plummets 80% in the severe scenario, 20% in the mild). For most other industries, the CBO saw a 10% drop in demand under the severe scenario, and a 3% fall under a mild scenario.

It's not all bad news. The healthcare sector of the economy will see demand for its services *increase* by 15% (severe) or 4% (mild). With one in three people falling ill, many of them requiring medication and hospitalization, it is little wonder that the "fortunes" of the health industry would rise as pandemic flu spreads.

Table 3: Assumed Declines in Demand by Industry, in the Event of an Avian Flu Pandemic

		Unit: percent	
		Severe Scenario	*Mild Scenario*
Private Industries	Agriculture	−10	−3
	Mining	−10	−3
	Utilities	0	0
	Construction	−10	−3
	Manufacturing	−10	−3
	Wholesale Trade	−10	−3
	Retail Trade	−10	−3
	Air Transportation	−67	−17

Table 3 – *cont'd*

		Unit: percent	
		Severe Scenario	*Mild Scenario*
Private Industries	Rail Transportation	−67	−17
	Transit	−67	−17
	Information (Published, broadcast)	0	0
	Finance	0	0
	Professional and Business Services	0	0
	Education	0	0
	Healthcare	+15	+4
	Arts and Recreation	−80	−20
	Accommodation	−80	−20
	Food Service	−80	−20
	Other Services (excluding government)	−5	−1
Government	Federal	0	0
	State and Local	0	0

Source: US Congressional Budget Office

Note: The severe scenario describes a pandemic that is similar to the 1918–19 Spanish flu outbreak. It incorporates the assumption that a particularly virulent strain of influenza infects 90 million people in the United States and kills more than two million of them. The mild scenario describes a pandemic that resembles the outbreaks of 1957–58 and 1968-69. It incorporates the assumption that 75 million people become infected in the US and about 100,000 of them die from the illness or complications.

On the supply side, the CBO estimates are somewhat more uniform across industries, (see Table 4). For nearly all sectors of the

US economy, 25% to 30% of the workforce will fall ill under severe and mild pandemic scenarios, respectively. The average worker will miss three weeks of work, although not all workers will be absent at the same time. Only the agricultural sector would have a degree of shelter from pandemics, the US government body said. The infection rate for farm workers will be one in 10 (severe), resulting in farmers missing an average of just one week of work. This is because most farm workers rarely need to come into contact with large numbers of people. But that may not hold true in other parts of the world, like Asia, where small farmers regularly market their produce directly to the end-consumer through wet markets and other outlets.

Table 4: Assumptions of Underlying Estimates of the Supply-Side Impact of an Avian Flu Pandemic

	Gross Attack Rate (Percent)		Weeks Out of Work		Case Fatality Rate (Percent)	
	Severe	Mild	Severe	Mild	Severe	Mild
Nonfarm Business	30	25	3.0	0.75	2.5	1.14
Farm	10	5	1.0	0.25	2.5	1.14
Household	30	25	3.0	0.75	2.5	1.14
Nonprofit Institution	30	25	3.0	0.75	2.5	1.14
Government	30	25	3.0	0.75	2.5	1.14

Source: US Congressional Budget Office

Note: The gross attack rate is the percentage of the population that is infected with a disease. The case fatality rate is the percentage of infected persons who eventually die from the disease or complications.

The CBO study provides insight into the impact of a flu pandemic on different industries. However, a number of caveats are in order. For one, the estimates are designed with the US economy in mind. In addition, the analysis only gives an indication of how demand might drop, or how many weeks a flu victim might be absent from work. While these are important indicators, useful to executives trying to gauge the impact of flu on their businesses, they do not paint the whole picture.

Most company business models include more complex factors than just labor supply and market demand. Companies rely on other firms to supply them with raw materials or services such as transportation and logistics. All companies, irrespective of whether they are in the manufacturing or service sector, need basic supplies of electric power and telecommunication services, including the internet. While the CBO saw no change in demand for utilities, for example, in all likelihood a pandemic could put demand pressure on electricity, water and other basic service providers. Simultaneously, electric power plant workers will fall sick at the same rate as the rest of society. Given a surge of demand and 30% drop in the labor force at utilities, most companies will be affected to some degree.

Clearly there is a need to consider how the fate of one industry—such as the transportation industry—can affect another. It is impossible to consider all the possible permutations and combinations. But individual managers charged with developing continuity plans for their businesses must factor in how all stakeholders in their business—employees, suppliers, consumers, even their suppliers' suppliers—might be affected by a flu pandemic. While this will differ greatly from industry to industry, all firms share a dependence on at least one thing—the proper functioning of basic infrastructure.

Cross-Cutting Infrastructure

On St. Valentine's Day 2006, Michael Osterholm, director of the Center for Infectious Disease Research and Policy at the University of Minnesota in Minneapolis, hosted a national summit on business planning for pandemic influenza.[5] Three hundred participants representing over 200 companies, including representatives of around

20 Fortune 50 companies, had signed up to hear the prognosis for business during and after the next pandemic flu. If the executives were expecting to be shocked into action, then they came to the right place. This was particularly true when the assembled panel of experts discussed how a flu pandemic might affect an economy's so-called "cross-cutting infrastructure"—electricity grids, the internet, telecommunication, transportation and shipping networks that form the backbone of a country's economy.

While the alarming picture the panelists painted referred primarily to the US economy, much of their commentaries could apply with equal force to other developed economies around the world. In the case of developing countries, where cross-cutting infrastructure is weak even at the best of times, it is hard to predict how a pandemic flu might affect the functioning of an economy. It could be argued that because businesses and citizens in these countries have greater experience in dealing with power shortages and inadequate infrastructure, any further deterioration brought about by pandemic flu would have little real impact on their economic fortunes.

For the audience of executives from the US, the message from the panelists was clear: companies and industries that provide a developed economy's backbone will suffer labor losses just like any other industry. This means that utilities, telecoms, internet service providers, like almost every other sector of the economy, will see at least a quarter of their employees fall ill and stay away from the workplace. And that doesn't even include those employees who may choose to stay home from work because they are terrified about catching flu at the office.

But according to the experts at the Minneapolis meeting, not all the "vertebrae" in an economy's infrastructural backbone are created equally. Some will be hit much harder than others. Companies that are using outdated equipment, or that are stretched under normal circumstances, will come under especially intense pressure in a pandemic. Similarly, if a service is labor intensive, then the provision of that service will be more affected by absenteeism.

Take electricity. Massoud Amin, director at the Center for the Development of Technological Leadership, also at the University of Minnesota, told the audience that the current electric-power supply sector in the US is already in deep trouble, without a pandemic flu.

"The system is already close to the edge," Amin said. At each and every level of the power-supply chain the American electricity grid is hurting, from tight supply of fuel sources needed to generate power, to the outdated machinery in power-generation plants. What's more, utility companies, like many other companies in other sectors of the US economy, have become so lean that "they have been downsized, right sized, and nearly capsized," Amin warned. Lean may make shareholders happy, but the impact on society could be disastrous if a quarter to a third of an already skeleton staff at such crucial companies are sick or skip work. And the power grid will be hard-pressed to cope with the erratic demand patterns for electricity that would persist through a flu pandemic.

Amin said it normally takes around two weeks to get the lights back on after a natural disaster such as Hurricane Katrina. These events are usually confined to geographic location and are, on the whole, one-off events. By definition, a pandemic would not be a localized event and would occur in multiple waves of six to eight weeks in length, making it far more challenging to keep power running smoothly.

It might be tempting to dismiss Amin's dire predictions, were it not for recent history. In August 2003, the US and Canada experienced their worst-ever electricity blackout. An estimated 40 million Americans and 10 million Canadians were left without power for a period of around 30 hours, resulting in an economic blow estimated at $6 billion. Water supplies in some areas were reportedly affected, the US rail company Amtrak was forced to stop some of its services, and factories were shut down. Laptop computer users were able to access the internet—until, that is, their computer batteries died.

Fellow panelist Marshall Sanders was more upbeat on the prospects for internet connectivity. Sanders is vice president for global security at Level3 Communications, a Colorado-based company that, according to the company website: "operates one of the largest communications and internet backbones in the world."[6]

Sanders said that the internet was designed to withstand a nuclear attack, and has demonstrated its resilience in the past, with the terror attacks of Sept. 11, 2001 being a case in point. But that is not to say companies can be complacent. Even if the internet remains robust, there are a host of other issues that can and should be addressed now. These include: remote access (Who is going to have it?); servers (Is there enough capacity to support a high number of employees working remotely?); and licenses for software (What numbers are required? When will they be purchased?).

But as Steven Ross, director of enterprise risk services for Deloitte & Touche in New York pointed out, scaring CEOs by proclaiming that the sky is falling won't help matters. Instead, he suggested that information-technology related pandemic-flu preparation be thought of as a means of improving worker productivity, regardless of whether a pandemic emerges or not. In the unfortunate event that a pandemic does occur, companies will still be covered. "We can manage this problem if we start now," Ross concluded.

Yet all the high-end IT in the world doesn't matter if goods can't be transported. On that front, Anne Marie Kappel, vice president of the World Shipping Council, had a less than encouraging view of the preparedness of businesses and the US economy in general to cope with disruptions in the shipping and transportation sectors. Like the electric-power industry, Kappel said that the transportation system — ports, road, rail — is plagued with tight capacity today.

Vessel capacity is available and would not really pose a problem because there would be little if any disruption to the operation of the ships at sea. However, land-side capacity is very tight, particularly in the US, and the operation of port facilities is labor intensive. This means that while cargo may move on ships it cannot reach its final destination without appropriate land-side support. Even today, tight capacity leads to delays and the problem will clearly be compounded should there be a loss of additional workers due to a flu pandemic.

"If we talk about a pandemic that will impact 25% to 35% of the workforce and you have an industry [like shipping] that is structured with billions of dollars of assets, none of which you can operate without people, [then] this will have an impact on the system," she warned.

Convincing healthy workers to come to work will be one of the biggest challenges for the transportation sector. It is not enough just to tell employees that they cannot get sick from the cargo. The message has to come from credible sources—from scientists, doctors and the government. "With Sars, we got the CDC to come out quickly and make public statements saying you could not get Sars from the cargo, which helped tremendously," Kappel noted.

* * * * * * * * * * * * * *

The challenge for the business community is to identify those areas that are within their scope of control and to take appropriate action now, while there is still time to prepare. Though costly and time consuming, developing a business continuity plan can help minimize the economic impact of a pandemic by anticipating disruption to infrastructure, absenteeism, a drop in demand for a company's goods or services, and a sharp drop in inputs from suppliers that will be equally affected by a pandemic.

The next section looks at examples of companies that have already embraced the concept of business continuity planning and are updating their plans to reflect pandemic flu scenarios.

Case Studies[7]

Hongkong and Shanghai Banking Corp. (HSBC)

When HSBC announced its pandemic flu plans in January 2006, it caused a stir in the business community. The world's number three bank predicts that 50% of its 253,000 employees could be absent from work during a flu pandemic. That figure is double the 25% to 35% that is commonly cited by the WHO, other international organizations, governments and even this book.

"None of us know the virulence of the virus, but I would rather be prepared for the worst," Bob Piggott, head of group crisis management for HSBC told the *Financial Times*.[8]

Jeremy Haworth, senior regional continuity planning manager for HSBC, said key issues for the bank are the following:

1. **Medical.** The company has consulted a panel of medical doctors to provide management with "sound advice" on the appropriateness of a number of proposed measures. The bank has offered free vaccinations for seasonal flu to its entire staff, with discounted jabs for their families. HSBC has also established an internal education campaign, including a dedicated website on the company's intranet. In addition, the bank has had a registered nurse train its staff on best health practices throughout the organization.

2. **Communications.** The bank has developed a communications web that stretches from its headquarters in London to Asia and

other regions. Haworth said the company is especially keen on building good surveillance and containment programs.

3. **Technology.** A main concern is the working arrangements for employees under a pandemic scenario. The bank is currently looking at technical issues related to providing staffers with the tools to work from home, from executive level down to the bank's "foot soldiers." Haworth said a key challenge is how to provide access to the bank's in-house computer systems from a remote location. HSBC in Hong Kong is also looking at split-site arrangements, and using its dedicated strategic recovery site which was built a couple of years ago in Hong Kong. In addition, the bank is preparing for an "inevitable increase" in customers' use of remote banking. The bank found that during Sars, few customers wanted to physically enter a bank, preferring instead to conduct their transactions through internet and phone banking. This will mean having to look carefully at server and call-center capacity issues in order to maintain the levels of service that customers have grown to expect.

Haworth urged companies to think carefully before drawing up a plan that hinges on the use of a single command center, since doing so could only serve to increase the chances of contamination of key decision makers:

"I recall during Sars the very first command center meeting we had," said Haworth. "We all sat down around the table and suddenly I realized it wasn't a good idea because all the decision makers were in the same room together." To avoid this, Haworth recommends that companies get used to holding such meetings remotely. "It takes a bit of getting used to but once you have conference call meetings, it actually works very effectively," he said.

Intel

Intel had first-hand experience with Sars when one of its employees in Hong Kong became infected with the disease in 2003.

The company occupied all of the 32nd floor and parts of the 25th and 29th floors of a central Hong Kong office block. The infected employee worked on the 32nd floor. When it discovered its employee had Sars, the firm shut down that floor for a week for thorough disinfection. Employees on the other floors were given the option to work from home, and many chose to do so. For Intel executives this wasn't too much of a problem, since they were used to working while on the road for business trips. But many support staff simply did not have the tools to work remotely. The company also put tight restrictions on travel, authorizing only business trips that were deemed urgent.

Jim Jeffs, senior attorney at Intel, said the company learned a lot from its experience with Sars—experience that is helping the firm plan for avian flu. "This time we are much more proactive," said Jeffs.

The company has come up with a regional plan to ensure it doesn't get caught off-guard again. This includes stockpiling essential supplies such as disinfectants for individuals, as well as for cleaning the office facilities. According to Jeffs, the company is not stockpiling antiviral drugs such as Tamiflu.

In addition, each of Intel's business groups has been tasked to draw up business continuity plans. In particular, the company's information technology group has been very active. During Sars, large numbers of people needed to access the company's servers from remote locations, and the system soon became overloaded. At that time, a note was sent to employees urging them to curtail their time online so as not to swamp the system. Since then, Intel has upgraded its IT network significantly in anticipation of a similar need for large numbers of its employees to work remotely in the future.

With some back-office operations located across the border in the mainland Chinese city of Shenzhen, the company has also factored in the possibility that either the Hong Kong or Beijing government might decide to seal its borders. If that were to happen, the company might need extra desk space in Hong Kong to accommodate returning managers seconded to the Shenzhen operations. Already, extra desks have been allocated to meet this need.

Jeffs said an important legal consideration is the privacy of an infected employee. During the Sars outbreak, Intel promptly reported the case to the authorities but made the decision to keep the employee's identity confidential in its internal communications.

Jeffs pointed out that Hong Kong laws, for example, require companies to take measures that are "reasonably practical" to ensure employee safety, but that these should be considered minimum standards. He said it is up to the executives in every company to consider from an ethical and moral standpoint: "Am I satisfied doing the minimum? Or do I feel more comfortable to do more to protect my employees than is absolutely required by the law?"

Hongkong Land

Hongkong Land is a major property investment, management and development group based in Hong Kong. The company's portfolio extends to about 5.5 million square feet of office and retail accommodation in 11 buildings in the Central area of Hong Kong, and another building in the Quarry Bay district of the territory. Of its roughly 650 clients, 50 come from the catering sector, including restaurants, cafès and bars—a sector of the economy that would be extremely sensitive to a pandemic flu. (In the case of the US economy, CBO predicts food service to witness an 80% drop in demand under a severe pandemic scenario and 20% under a mild one.)

Hugh Andrew, senior asset manager of commercial property in Hong Kong for the company, estimated that up to 60,000 people work in Hongkong Land buildings each day, and another 120,000 visit the properties.

"That's 180,000 people, or 3% of the population of Hong Kong," Andrew said "We take that responsibility very seriously in how we might be impacting what goes on here should there be an outbreak of avian flu."

Andrew said the company's business continuity planning governs two areas: the continuity of Hongkong Land itself; and the provision of services to assist Hongkong Land's tenants so that they can carry on with business.

Andrew had developed a simulation model which showed that if up to 70% of its operations team became incapacitated, the company could still function. But if 30% of its management were out sick, services in some buildings may have to be reduced, and some buildings even closed down.

He said the procedures that were established during Sars allowed the company to devise a procedure whereby it can isolate separate teams to ensure that coverage is available.

"Fundamentally, we can create 11 or 12 'mini' Hongkong Lands in each of our buildings," explained Andrew. "They are allowed to make decisions and run their operations in isolation."

Andrew said a critical element in the company's strategy for pandemic flu prevention is hygiene, both in the home and the workplace. His company's plan has four stages.

Stage 1:   Awareness and preparedness, including purchasing the necessary supplies and equipment, and training staff.

Stage 2:   When a case of avian flu in humans is recorded in Hong Kong.

Stage 3:   When a case of avian flu in humans is recorded in a property belonging to Hongkong Land's portfolio. In the same way it is important for the landlord to inform the tenant of any developments, tenants must resist the temptation to avoid negative publicity and keep the landlord informed of any suspected outbreaks.

Stage 4:   When human-to-human transmission triggers a pandemic. "I don't have a detailed contingency for that because frankly nobody [does]," said Andrew. "The important element of our planning would be to be flexible and ready to adjust to the threat as it changes and affects what we're doing."

Morgan Stanley Asia

As the chief administrative officer for Morgan Stanley Asia, Alexandria Albers' job includes developing contingency plans and crisis management for the investment bank's operations in Asia. With more than 10 years experience of working in the region, Albers is drawing on the knowledge she gained during the Sars crisis to build a business continuity plan for pandemic flu.

During the 2003 crisis, Morgan Stanley's goal was to balance and manage employee safety and the firm's desire to continue to service clients. The company did this through:

1. Maintaining open, regular dialogue with employees. Albers said that maintaining daily communication with employees was

probably the most important component of the company's Sars plan. At one point the firm conveyed important medical information via a web cast to 55,000 employees worldwide. This had a "tremendous effect" on reducing the anxiety level of company personnel and the company would certainly do that again in the event of a pandemic flu, she said.

2. Seeking professional advice. The company regularly consulted with doctors and others in the medical profession.
3. Remaining globally connected. It was important that the company spoke with one voice, both internally and externally.
4. Responding quickly. Albers said it was critical that the firm created a decision-making group to deal with the issues as they arose.

Albers considered the current situation for pandemic flu to be different from Sars in two important ways. First, companies clearly have more time to prepare. Morgan Stanley has had an avian-flu task force in place since early 2005. This has given the company a valuable opportunity to stress test different scenarios. Second, employees are much better informed about avian flu than Sars, thanks to extensive coverage in the media and efforts by governments and the medical community to educate the public.

Yet pandemic flu is also fundamentally different from the catastrophic events that most crisis managers are trained to handle. It's not simply a case of a breakdown in the firm's computer system or the loss of access to a mission-critical premise. Instead, it will be a company's human resources—its people—that will be unavailable.

Albers said it is critical that third-party vendors also have robust plans in place, particularly suppliers of infrastructure such as telecoms and technology providers. Governments should also ensure that the infrastructure is resilient to stresses and not leave the entire business continuity planning responsibility with the private sector.

For now the firm is stepping up its inhouse efforts to keep staff informed of the latest developments by setting up a dedicated web page on the company's intranet. It is also recommending its employees worldwide to get shots for seasonal flu.

In the event of an outbreak, the company would restrict travel to and from affected areas, but would seek guidance from global health organizations before taking action. Morgan Stanley has a "direct line" to the WHO in order to understand how best the company should prepare for a pandemic and to stay informed real time. Albers said the company would consider relocating critical staff to other sites and would take steps to restrict gatherings and increase the use of video and audio conferencing.

"We feel that good communication is key to keeping our people healthy and our business going," Albers noted.

Cisco Systems Asia Pacific

Dominic Scott, principal consultant, public sector with Cisco Systems Asia Pacific, said his company has also learned a lot from Sars as well as from the Boxing Day tsunami about how important the role a company's network can play during a disaster. Scott believed there were five information-technology related questions executives should ask:

1. Are employees able to work from home or some other remote location?
2. Can the company communicate effectively with employees, customers and business partners during times of crisis?
3. Does the company have the ability to set up remote offices or temporary facilities with minimal disruption to its core business?

4. Does the company have a systems-wide approach to physical security and information security?
5. Are there backup systems in place?

In the case of Cisco employees, most are now equipped with access to VPNs, or virtual private networks, and other tools which allow them to work from any location that offers broadband. While this sometimes entails subsidizing employees' home broadband costs, the goal is to offer employees access to the same functionalities at home as they would have in the office.

Another tool that Cisco uses is mass voicemail messaging. This allows the CEO, or any other senior executive, to send a voice mail directly into the voice mail box of all Cisco employees worldwide within a matter of hours. This is a good way for sharing important information with employees, whether it is quarterly results or urgent information during a crisis.

Scott also believed it is vital that companies pay close attention to security issues. Cisco monitors all offices worldwide using IP video-surveillance cameras. This allows the company's senior executives to see what is going on in any office anywhere around the world in real time.

Scott urged managers to consider business continuity planning from a broad perspective:

"IT and network infrastructure can play an important role for emergencies like Sars or terrorism," he said. "And the strategies that [companies] put in place also have the potential to give quite a few business benefits beyond simply coping with that emergency."

Conclusions
The potential impact of a pandemic flu will differ from industry to industry. At the heart of the issue will be absenteeism. Most estimates

put the range of absenteeism rates from 25% to 35%. Some corporations are using higher estimates for the business continuity plans. HSBC, for example, estimated that 50% of its workforce could be affected by a pandemic.

Yet not all the challenges are internal. Companies must also consider the effects a pandemic will have on their suppliers, their business partners and how the demand for their goods or services will be affected.

Executives have to give serious consideration to how the cross-cutting infrastructure such as electric power, the internet, telecoms, and shipping and transportation might cope with the effects of a pandemic.

After factoring in these elements, companies should devise a business continuity plan that is suitable for their business. This chapter highlights how some of the bigger companies are tackling the problem. What can smaller companies that don't have access to the same resources as global corporations do to prepare for a pandemic? The following chapter takes a closer look at the elements of business continuity planning and offers suggestions to help managers jump-start the process.

The Impact of Sars on Cathay Pacific Airways

Within the short space of a few weeks, Hong Kong airline Cathay Pacific Airways saw its daily passenger numbers plummet from 35,000 to as low as 5,330 as a result of the Sars outbreak. The airline was forced to suspend half its flights, and parked 22 of its fleet, which in 2003 was made up of around 85 aircraft. What follows is an account of how Cathay Pacific survived the Sars pandemic.

Note: Taken from a speech given by Cathay Pacific's Alan Wong, general manager, corporate communications, to a gathering of Hong Kong civil servants in May 2004.

Crisis Development

Without a doubt, Sars was the worst commercial challenge ever faced by the airline. It affected not only the airline but the whole of Hong Kong: flights and hotels and other tourism-related facilities were virtually empty.

During the height of the crisis, literally a handful of passengers flying from Los Angeles, Frankfurt or Vancouver was not uncommon. There was one flight we operated to Taipei that had only one booking, and on the day even that passenger didn't show.

The alarm about Sars was first raised on 12 March [2003] when 26 medical staff were taken ill in Hanoi, Vietnam. Within a week 219 cases were reported in different parts of the world.

Sars first became an issue for Cathay Pacific on 16 March when the airline was informed that a passenger who had flown with us to Canada 10 days previously had been taken ill.

Airlines probably face more crises than any other business. However, handling Sars did not appear in any crisis-management textbook. First of all, very little was known about it, how it was transmitted and, although clearly deadly, did it pose a sweeping danger to public health, let alone our airline?

Even though the facts had not yet been established, intuition told us that whatever Sars was, it had the potential to be an enormous problem for the airline.

Crisis Response

With so little information you can imagine that we had very little to go on to structure our response. But as with any crisis, we were able to break it down into three basic components: Response, Reassurance and Recovery.

The initial response of course needs to be quick. News about the Cathay Pacific passenger who may have had Sars came to us on a Sunday. We issued a news release that day headlined: "Cathay Pacific initiates precautions against Sars…"

…The very next morning, the airline put together a dedicated team of senior representatives from all operational departments, and headed by a company director to manage the situation. They held daily briefings to assess developments and create action plans for the duration of the Sars crisis at 7:30 every morning.

At the beginning, no one had a clear idea of the dimensions of Sars and the issues we therefore faced. But it was clear that our first concern was to protect the health of our passengers and staff.

There were no minimal recommendations for airlines to deal with the situation, so we devised our own. We immediately posted notices at check-in counters detailing World Health Organization guidelines and Sars symptoms. Staff—particularly those who come into contact with customers—and therefore at greater potential risk, were also advised.

Health updates from our own medical services team were provided to all staff on a daily basis via newsletters, notices and advice posted on the airline's intranet system, which all staff have access to all over the world.

Fairly soon, it became obvious that we were to face very serious commercial implications. Passengers stopped flying in droves. The WHO placed a travel ban on Hong Kong. Cathay Pacific started to lose $3 million a day and the company issued its first ever profit warning. In short, the crisis became one of the company's survival.

To illustrate just how fast this situation came upon us, on March 6, the company announced its second best ever profit for the year

2002. Ten days later we received our Sars alert, and within a month the profit warning was issued at the Hong Kong Stock Exchange.

In this situation our objectives shifted toward conserving cash, preserving jobs and maintaining the integrity of our network. Effective internal communication was paramount. Our chief executive, David Turnbull, convened a meeting with senior managers. His address was filmed and sent to ports as well. His message was direct: "We must save money so that we might live to fight another day."

We cancelled almost half of our services and parked 22 aircraft. Yet we kept our network intact. When US carriers quit Hong Kong, we maintained services so that Hong Kong could maintain contact with the outside world, and people who need to travel to do business could still do so.

Management cancelled all non-critical projects, deferred major capital expenditure, shareholders voted to accept a 50% cut in their 2002 final dividend and staff—more than 99% of them—volunteered to take a period of unpaid leave. Early on, the company said that it would do everything possible to save jobs. It was this promise that brought staff on our side. And not one member of the Hong Kong [team] suffered the loss of a job.

Reassuring the Public

Once we understood the real situation, we had to let people know that it was indeed safe to fly. The main issue was whether Sars was a health issue or an aviation issue. We had to struggle against press headlines that initially called Sars the "jet flu." We needed to reassure people that although people may have arrived sick in places— promoting Sars' global spread—people were not getting sick on aircraft. This misperception was growing so great that we had to speak up for ourselves.

Our "Flying Without Fear" campaign was launched in April.

Advertisements were placed in newspapers describing the many measures we had taken, and our frequent customers were sent individual letters to answer their concerns. We organized press tours on our aircraft and had them meet with engineers who were able to show how air within an aircraft is kept almost as clean as a hospital operating theater.

Food was sealed in our flight kitchens so that people would have confidence about hygiene, even though Sars was at no time transmitted in food. We also worked with the [Hong Kong] Civil Aviation Department, the global aviation industry group IATA, and the travel trade.

Our website was updated with the latest World Health Organization information and recommendations daily.

Recovery from the Crisis

To every crisis there is a recovery. Throughout Sars, it wasn't just Cathay Pacific that was suffering; so was Hong Kong. With tourists and business travelers turning away in droves, we had to do something to help ourselves as well as the economy. So we created the Hong Kong Tourism Coalition, an ad-hoc grouping of tourism-related industries that included hotels, tour companies and airlines, and we launched the "We Love Hong Kong" campaign.

The campaign was initially to last one month. It lasted three. During the original Tourism Coalition phase in May, some 1,300 travel agents and 80 hotels enrolled and airlines contributed 30,000 discount tickets. Cathay Pacific donated more than 8,000 tickets itself, all of which we redeemed. More than 10,000 taxi drivers also got behind the campaign.

After Hong Kong was declared Sars free we restored 70% of our flights by the end of August and all flights and aircraft were back by the end of September.

Insurance industry

If you are worried your company will take a heavy financial hit from a pandemic flu, spare a thought for the insurance industry.

According to Steven Weisbart, economist with the Insurance Information Institute, a severe flu pandemic along the lines of the Spanish flu of 1918 could cost the US life insurers $133 billion in additional death claims. A moderate flu pandemic similar to the Asian flu of 1957-58 and the Hong Kong flu of 1968-69 would cost $31 billion in additional claims.

The institute says that normally flu hits either the very old or very young. But in the case of a pandemic, all bets are off. In 1918 the highest number of deaths was recorded in the 25-34 age group, a demographic that, the institute says "has significant individual life insurance in force."

The institute says that a future flu pandemic could be even more damaging to the insurance industry's fortunes for a number of reasons. First, there is the issue of immunity. In 1918 it is plausible that some of the people over 65 had acquired some immunity from their exposures to earlier flu strains. If the next pandemic flu turns out to be H5 linked, then today's elderly would not have any immunity. Second, the absolute number of elderly is greater today than it was in 1918 (this is true for the population in general as well).

However, post-pandemic could bring better news for insurers.

"If the example of 1918 is any guide, in the year following the pandemic, a record number of people would apply for new life insurance policies, vividly convinced of the value of the protection," Weisbart said.

Endnotes

1   Reprinted by permission of *Foreign Affairs*, "Preparing for the Next Pandemic," Michael T. Osterholm, July/August 2005. Copyright 2005 by the Council on Foreign Relations, Inc.

2   See http://www.iata.org/pressroom/industry_facts/fact_sheets/economic_social_benefits.htm

3   See http://www.adb.org/Documents/News/2003/nr2003065.pdf

4   "A Potential Influenza Pandemic: Possible Macroeconomic Effects and Policy Issues," The Congress of the United States Congressional Budget Office, Dec. 8, 2005

5   Reporting from Minneapolis was provided by Emily Zylla who attended the Business Planning for Pandemic Influenza: A National Summit, Feb 14 -15, 2006. The event was hosted by the University of Minnesota's Center for Infectious Disease Research and Policy (CIDRAP), and co-sponsored by the US Chamber of Commerce and the Minnesota Chamber of Commerce.

6   See www.level3.com

7   The case studies contained herein are based on presentations made by executives to two gatherings devoted to pandemic flu organized by the American Chamber of Commerce in Hong Kong in November 2005 and February 2006.

8   "HSBC warns on possible bird flu toll—Estimates dwarf government and WHO figures," by Andrew Jack, *Financial Times*, Jan. 10, 2006

Chapter Six

So What's the Plan?

It should have been a legal nightmare when an explosion in a US-owned refinery in Belize sent toxic chemicals through the air, affecting workers and residents in the surrounding area. The company had a computer-controlled alarm system, but it failed to work. Yet when claimants sued, jurors came out in favor of the management of the refinery. This was despite the fact that the premises' computerized alarm system had clearly failed to work at the time of the explosion.

How did a company with a defective disaster-response system manage to get off the hook? The reason is simple, according to Cheryl Falvey, an attorney with Akin Gump Strauss Hauer and Field LLP based in Washington, DC.

"Most jurors understand that accidents happen, that human error can occur and that processes don't always work the way they were planned to," explained Falvey, speaking at a business pandemic flu planning seminar in Minneapolis in February 2006.

On the other hand, juries will not forgive, and will punish companies that fail to assess a problem in advance, or neglect to commit the necessary resources to deal with it. Furthermore, juries are equally unimpressed by companies that fail to bring the problem to the attention of senior management.

Behind juries' unrelenting stance is the concept of "foreseeability." In other words, could a company have reasonably anticipated an event—such as an explosion in a chemical plant? If so, did the company take the appropriate measures to prevent the event or mitigate its consequences?

In the case of the refinery in Belize, the company had gone to great lengths to prevent explosions and had comprehensive policies in place to minimize damage should one occur. It had conducted environmental impact studies; carried out emergency response drills with local officials; trained doctors in the local hospitals on how to treat victims of chemical explosions; and installed a state-of-the-art computerized alarm system.

So even though the alarm system ultimately failed, the company could produce documented evidence that it had conducted monthly tests on the alarm. Moreover, other policies the company had in place were sufficient to demonstrate to jurors that the company had "foreseen" a potential problem and had prepared for that threat appropriately.

Of course, the question arises: What constitutes "foreseeability?" Falvey said the concept of what is foreseeable and what is not is a highly fluid one. The most important determinant, however, is whether adequate, accurate and authoritative scientific information on the scope of risks a company faces exist. If there is, then the event will probably be considered "foreseeable" and companies will be judged accordingly.

In the case of pandemic flu, there is a huge body of scientific material that clearly points to a real threat if not directly from H5N1 then from another flu virus at some point in the future. Should an employee decide to sue for personal injury, or a customer because of a company's failure to meet its contractual obligations, then the onus could be on the company to show that they assessed the risk properly and took reasonable steps to prevent or mitigate its impact. Falvey said this could include providing information to the courts on budget spending and may require a deposition from the CEO in order to show the degree of seriousness the company attached to the problem prior to the event. Any decision not to take action would need to be based on economic or engineering decisions that were made (and documented) at that time. Post-hoc rationalizations of why a company did not act just won't fly, Falvey said.

The implications are crystal clear: having a business continuity plan for pandemic flu is not optional. Not only does it make good sense for running a business during a flu crisis, it could also save a company's hide when the dust has settled and management is called to account for its actions (or inaction) during the pandemic.

* * * * * * * * * * * * * *

Perhaps the most fundamental question executives need to consider before launching into planning for a pandemic is whether there is top management support for the idea. Jeremy Haworth of HSBC said much of the initiative behind the bank's pandemic planning came from the top. And because it is a priority from on high it has become a priority for Haworth and all the bank's planning staff in the Asian region.

Yet while Newton and Haworth have supportive senior management, there is one slight difference. In Newton's case, her headquarters called on her to handle it because she is in Asia. However, there is danger in this approach.

As Richard Martin, an analyst with Australia-based consulting firm International Market Assessment Asia writes:[1]

> "Companies that start down the Asia-only path realize within a few weeks that a pandemic business continuity plan can only be undertaken as a global project but these first few misdirected weeks can be quite frustrating for the Asia team."

Martin said senior management must get involved because, as the name suggests, a pandemic flu will impact the whole world as it spreads in successive, potentially lethal waves. This means that global business results—including sales growth and profitability—will be affected. Provisions for this scenario need to be included in any business continuity plan worth the paper it is written on. Since only top management can sign off on changes in mission-critical parameters, then it follows that management must throw its weight fully behind any pandemic planning, Martin added.

That said, Craig Foster, senior executive vice president with risk consulting firm Hill & Associates, said that since Asia has been and likely will be the epicenter of a pandemic, there is some logic on the part of companies that decide to make their Asian operations into "centers of excellence" for battling pandemic flu.

As H5N1 spreads, moving into India, the Middle East, Europe and eventually (some say) to the US, this perception should change. However, two surveys suggest that Asia is still leading the way on pandemic preparedness. One survey[2] by the American Chamber of Commerce in Hong Kong, showed that close to 60% of the 80 companies surveyed said they had a "clearly stated plan" for handling avian influenza. It should be noted that companies surveyed were in attendance at a conference on pandemic flu planning and as such probably display a higher interest in the topic than other companies. Even so, a similar survey conducted in the US by the Deloitte Center for Health Solutions[3]—part of professional services firm Deloitte & Touche USA—showed that planning for a flu pandemic still has a long way to go to capture the attention of American executives. Of the 179 completed responses received from large American companies, a total of two thirds either disagreed or strongly disagreed with the statement: "My company has adequately planned ways to protect itself from the effects of a human avian influenza breakout."

The Deloitte report goes on to conclude that many of the companies surveyed are taking a "wait-and-see attitude." Part of the reason seems to be a belief that a miracle vaccine will appear that will wipe out the threat of pandemic flu in one easy swipe. This would save companies time, money and efforts on "wasteful" pandemic planning activities. And it would provide many around the world with the chance to gloat at all the scaremongers and say: "I told you so!"

However, waiting for a vaccine is unwise as there is a very long way to go before a reliable one without any nasty side effects—that is effective against the strain of flu virus that triggers the next pandemic (remember, it does not have to be the H5N1 strain)—can be efficiently produced in the volumes needed, and that can be distributed properly to the world's population. Similarly, doubts remain about the usefulness of antiviral drugs in preventing or controlling a pandemic.

Hill & Associate's Foster agreed: "Any focus on antivirals as a panacea is folly and only addresses one part of risk management strategies and business continuity measures that will be necessary to respond effectively and recover efficiently from a pandemic."

In the absence of any guarantees, the only certainty is that a plan is better than no plan.

Decisions, Decisions

The most important thing executives must recognize from the outset is that pandemic planning is different from other forms of business continuity planning. Yet most experts agree that a company's plan for pandemic flu should be consistent with a company's business continuity plan that covers other disaster scenarios.

Many companies, especially those in the financial sector, have long had sophisticated plans to deal with a wide range of scenarios ranging from terrorism to natural disasters to breakdown of critical systems or equipment. Yet the focus has been on data recovery, and setting up alternative work facilities that are spread over a wider geographic area. Traditionally—and especially in the world of finance and banking—these backup plans have been driven by a firm's IT department.

Under a pandemic flu scenario, people—not premises—will be threatened most. The impact will not only be internal—as might be the case if a company's offices are ravaged by fire—but will be external as well. Besides employees, the pandemic will affect customers, suppliers, business partners and employees' families.

The IT element of a business continuity plan cannot be ignored, but that still does not change the fact that with pandemic flu, perhaps more than under any other business continuity planning scenario, the focus will be squarely on people.

Predicted rates of absenteeism for a pandemic flu range from the conservative low single digit figure to the more commonly quoted 25% to 35%. Some organizations consider these figures to be too low. HSBC is basing its plans on the much higher absenteeism rate of 50%. The number of employees that fail to report to work may bear little relation to actual infection rates for the flu—fear of infection, the need to take care of children if schools close or to care for ill relatives—a number of factors could compound the problem. As past experience shows, pandemics hit in waves and can take two years to pass. Figure 2 shows how one model predicts levels of absenteeism during an eight-week wave of pandemic flu. In this case, the New Zealand government suggests that employers should make plans to operate with only 85% of staff for the duration of the pandemic period, but that during the peak of a pandemic, staffing levels could drop to as low as 50%.

For an organization, absent employees mean a compromised skill set. For some industries, such as banking and insurance, those left holding the fort may have to handle even greater workloads than normal. During Sars, many banking customers opted to conduct their transactions via online or telephone banking. During a pandemic flu, will there be enough staff to handle the surge in call volume? Are mega call centers advisable under pandemic conditions where gatherings of large numbers of people in one place may serve only to invite further calamity?

The first, and perhaps the most difficult decision executives must face, is to identify which employees and which jobs are critical so that the company can continue to function. This is not as straightforward as it first appears, since few employees like to be considered peripheral.

Figure 2: Total Attack Rate 50% Over 8 Weeks, Using the FluAid Model (New Zealand case)

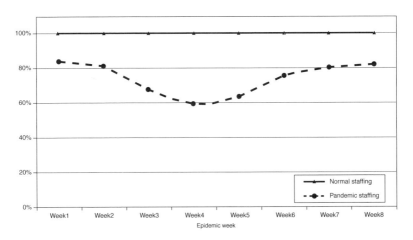

Source: Ministry of Economic Development, New Zealand, October 2005.
© Crown Copyright

Companies that already have business continuity plans for other scenarios should already have identified key employees or the "chosen few" as one commentator calls them, as well as the skill sets needed to keep the business running. For these companies, this first step in pandemic planning should not pose a problem.

For every industry, and maybe even each company, the decision as to what functions are essential and who can perform these functions will differ. On this count, there are few external sources or guidelines that will help in the selection. It is up to the management of each company to make these difficult but important decisions.

There is some debate as to whether employees should be informed of their status. Most business continuity planning advisors encourage managers to do so since this means people will be mentally prepared to carry out their roles and can jump into action without any delay once the pandemic plan has been triggered. These decisions should be made on the basis of a company's own corporate culture. The same selection of critical/noncritical staff will have to be done for company plants and offices, as well as for suppliers, and service providers.

Foster from Hill & Associates considered the issue of suppliers to be a "mission critical" one. "[For] multinational corporations that rely on outsourcing...their contingency planning is potentially only as strong as the weakest link in what are often very extended supply chains that rely on third, fourth and fifth parties."

The good news is that once some of these sensitive issues are addressed, the whole pandemic planning process becomes considerably easier. This is partly because there is a growing body of external sources of information available to help managers navigate subsequent stages of business continuity planning, including a host of government and private-sector websites offering templates and generic tools, to risk-consulting firms offering tailored advice on business planning for pandemic flu.

The Elements of a Pandemic Plan

While turning to outside help for devising a business continuity plan is always a possibility, there is no reason why one cannot be drawn up inhouse. In fact, it is preferable that it is devised within the business since a company's own employees should know best the organization's needs as well as its strengths and weaknesses. Wherever possible, companies should draw from existing business continuity plans but should bear in mind the fundamental differences of a pandemic from other disasters and modify accordingly. Table 5 lists some of the main attributes of a pandemic flu that make it different from a more "typical" disaster, as understood by the New Zealand government.

It is advisable to appoint an inhouse "influenza manager," supported by a team from selected departments, and charge them with building a plan. Since members of this team are equally susceptible to the flu virus as any other employee, substitute team members should also be identified. Additional members from outside the organization including medical advisors or communications professionals could also be appointed to supplement the team.

The team should understand the goals and objective of the plan: To mitigate the risk of a pandemic flu outbreak on the business so that it can continue to function as best as possible. This needs to be done while maximizing the safety of employees. In addition to activities during a pandemic, the plan should also consider actions that should be taken pre- and post-pandemic. Pre-pandemic planning is arguably the most important part of the pandemic plan. Proper development of this part of the plan is critical to the successful

Table 5: Comparing a Pandemic with a More Typical Disaster

Notice	It is quite likely that there will be some advance warning from the development of the pandemic overseas, but it is always possible that any warning period may be very short. Should pandemic influenza spread within New Zealand it will probably be some weeks before the full impact on workforce will be felt, although there may be some early impacts resulting from closures of schools and similar containment measures.
Primary Effect:	Unlike natural disasters, where any disruption to business service provision is likely to be hardware-related, disruption to business operation in the event of a pandemic is anticipated to be mainly human-resource oriented. [New Zealand's] Ministry of Health advises that businesses should plan for up to 50% staff absences for periods of about two weeks at the height of a severe pandemic wave, and lower levels of staff absence for a few weeks either side of the peak. Overall a pandemic wave may last about eight weeks. Note that the pandemic may come in waves of varying severity over time.

Source: New Zealand Ministry of Economic Development, © Crown Copyright, 2005

execution of the rest of the plan during the pandemic and post-pandemic stages.

1. People

Armed with a decisive list of critical and non-critical functions, the first task at hand is to ensure that all essential roles have a backup or "understudy", who can step in to fill the role should the main actors fall ill or become unavailable for work. This may seem like an overwhelming challenge, after all, how can a bank's star trader be replaced by a junior staff member? The goal here is to keep the functions of the position ticking over in the absence of the trader. This may be for a relatively short period of say, 10 days, until the absent banker returns. Most likely, there will be people who can step up to the plate and fill a bigger role, especially if it is only for a limited period of time. However, in the case that nobody exists to fill a role, then the pandemic planning team should raise an alarm flag and take action as soon as possible. These actions should include cross-training or skills training for staff so that a greater pool of employees is available to perform critical functions.

Separating workers into autonomous or semiautonomous teams ahead of a pandemic allows teams to work physically apart from each other, thus minimizing risk of cross-contamination. But it should be borne in mind that this only minimizes the risk of infection while employees are at work. Controlling employee interactions outside of the workplace is an entirely different matter, and for most purposes, impossible to achieve.

The pandemic planning team, together with the human resources department, may have to devise reporting policies that reflect the new (albeit temporary) organizational structure and operating environment. Some policy areas that will need to be addressed early on in the pandemic planning process include the issues of working from home and sick leave.

It is important that employees take seriously the company's request for them to stay at home if they feel ill. This must be communicated clearly to staff members at all stages of the pandemic, but especially in the pre-pandemic stage.

One reason why staff might be tempted to turn up to work even if they feel ill is because of ambiguous company policies regarding leave. Companies should outline in advance its policies for sick leave, paid and unpaid leave as they relate specifically to pandemic flu. Local labor laws will play a role here, but companies should consider going beyond the minimum required by law and demonstrate a degree of flexibility on these issues.

For international companies with overseas operations, special consideration may need to be given to expatriate staff, some of whom may demand repatriation in a time of crisis. A word of warning: during the Sars crisis, some companies were accused by their local employees of giving expatriate staff preferential treatment. Care should be taken to avoid this situation as it has a long-term potential to destroy team spirit. Risk consultant Foster said that many companies have learned their lesson in this regard. "Today's contingency plans are [more] 'inclusive' and often extend benefits such as allowances or alternative accommodation to key local executives."

For international companies or companies where employees travel extensively, the travel policy and procedures will need to be reviewed. Many companies said they will instigate travel restrictions should a pandemic occur. This may entail the introduction of a special approval system for travel whereby only urgent business trips are approved. Some travel service providers offer software that allows companies to keep track of employees' whereabouts while on overseas business trips. Airline, hotel and schedule details from the travel reservation are captured by the software and presented in an easy-to-view way that allows managers to pinpoint the location of employees at any given time. This can reduce the time taken to locate employees in the event of an emergency, or a change in the pandemic flu alert levels. (Many MNCs already have such systems in place in light of the increased risk from terrorism.) Again, these measures would only cover business travel. Companies may also wish to monitor employee vacation travel, although this would require the consent of employees.

Of course, all this assumes that airlines will continue to operate. In Chapter 5, the Cathay Pacific case study showed that the airline continued to operate even though many flights were almost empty. In the event of a flu pandemic, airlines may not have the luxury of this choice if authorities decide to ban international travel. Business continuity plans should consider these kinds of external factors, too, since they have a potential to considerably disrupt business activities.

And, in a world where just-in-time delivery is the name of the game, disruption to a company's supply chain could also be significant. As such, sharing continuity plans with critical suppliers is a must. "A risk assumed by one, is a risk imposed on all," said Foster.

2. Information Technology & Security

The internet and other technologies will provide a vital lifeline for businesses during a pandemic crisis. Yet many continuity plans are based on the assumption of normal power supplies. But is that a safe assumption? Cross-critical infrastructure, including power supply, is particularly vulnerable to disruption by extraordinary events such as a pandemic. Similarly, telecommunications networks could be overloaded or even rationed in the event of a severe pandemic.

In the same way, a company should define critical employees and critical suppliers, the pandemic planning team should also prioritize the company's different systems. These core systems should be strengthened and backed up regularly to ensure stable and secure access at all times.

Modifying inhouse systems to enable access from a remote location poses its own set of problems. This is one of the headaches for banks like HSBC which is currently grappling with finding ways for its foot soldiers to access the bank's inhouse system from their homes or other locations. Technological considerations aside, the security implications of such a move are enormous.

For some companies there will be systems that cannot be performed through remote access. In this case, these companies may have to rely on the split site solutions. If this is the case, then companies should consider investing to ensure that such facilities are as "infection free" as possible.

For most companies, the main challenge will be to make sure their systems are robust enough to deal with the extra traffic generated by more employees accessing the network from home. Some are now taking steps to increase the capacity of their servers and have introduced schemes to encourage employees to install broadband. Companies will need to consider if they wish to expand the number of employees that have remote access. This will entail significant investment as additional purchases of laptops and software licenses will be required.

Companies may wish to consider building in advance online web portals or bulletin boards that would allow self-reporting by employees. This would facilitate better communication between employees as it makes it easier to know the whereabouts of team members and reduce over-reliance on email.

Security issues should also be considered. As Hurricane Katrina showed, at times of social unrest, looting is not uncommon. Warehouses storing food and medical supplies could be especially vulnerable at times of crisis. Hiring additional security personnel may be challenging if pandemic flu infection rates are high.

3. Legal Issues

In the opening of this chapter attorney Cheryl Falvey described perhaps a main legal consideration for developing a pandemic flu business continuity plan: to protect a company from legal action post-pandemic. This section expands further on this and other themes related to legal liability and pandemic flu. According to Falvey, a company's failure to take reasonable action before, during and after a flu pandemic could result in it being sued by a third party who felt he or she had been injured in some way by a company's negligence; or a supplier that considered the company to be in breach of contract; or an employee who believed the company had violated labor laws. Take for example a company's obligations to shareholders. Since shareholders make important investment decisions based on the companies' public statements, it is important that all such statements can be backed up with hard evidence. If a company tries to allay investor fear by saying it intends to use alternative suppliers should a pandemic strike existing suppliers and render them inoperable, then the company must be able to show that it has taken concrete action to identify and secure alternative suppliers. In the world of legal liability, intentions alone are not sufficient.

For contract issues, companies should not expect to be able to invoke automatically *force majeure*—literally "greater force," a clause often included in contracts that limits liability arising from natural or unforeseen catastrophes that inhibit a party to the contract from fulfilling its obligations. *Force majeure* will not apply if there were reasonable actions a company could have taken which could have prevented a breach of contract, Falvey said. For example, since the 1970s, terrorism and hijacking have been considered under the law as "foreseeable" events, and the onus is on airlines to take appropriate measures to prevent them or minimize the impact of such attacks. If companies act now, there might still be scope for modifying contracts to provide clauses that would cover failure to meet obligations due to a flu pandemic (or indeed other types of pandemics), Falvey suggested.

Another significant area of concern in pandemic planning is the legal liabilities companies face in the more operational areas of the business. What is a company's legal obligation to its staff should a pandemic flu strike? Can a company tell its employees to go home, or prevent a suspected flu carrier from entering its premises? Is a company obliged to pay salaries and provide other benefits during a pandemic? These are just some of the more specific legal issues that a company needs to consider when drawing up its business continuity plans. Table 6 summarizes some of the main legal issues facing employers in the US as seen by law firm Littler Mendelson.

4.   Communications

A watertight communications strategy is probably one of the most critical aspects of a business continuity plan for pandemic flu. In fact, some experts would argue that effective communications and an efficient medium of communications as *the* most critical elements of the plan. If past pandemics have taught us anything it is that panic and fear can push people to overreact and behave irrationally compared to the actual threat posed by the disease. Effective communication with employees, customers, suppliers and business partners can alleviate fear substantially and reduce the chances of irrational reactions. The way we communicate risk is of vital importance, said Thomas Abraham, director of the public health media program at the University of Hong Kong's Journalism and Media Studies Centre. Abraham said the average person takes the opinions of experts and interprets them based on his or her interpretation of reality. That is why people are more afraid of dying from a shark attack than a heart attack, despite the fact that the chances of dying from cardiac arrest are considerably higher in most countries. In the case of avian flu, this process of risk communication, or accurately conveying risk to the general public, has been particularly bad, said Abraham. "We really need to understand risk communication and put it into practice. That really is the bottom line," he said.

* * * * * * * * * * * * * *

Table 6: Main Legal Considerations for US Employers

Compensation, Leave, Benefits and Labor Relations Worries	In the event that a severe pandemic reaches the US, as much as 40% of a company's workforce may be out sick at any given time. With no preparedness plan or communicable illness policy in place, employers would be unprepared to meet staffing and operational needs, or adjust benefits and compensation plans for employees who exceed allotted days of leave. Employers might also trigger labor contract restrictions if they use contract employees or re-hire retirees, or may suffer adverse and long-term employee relations harm by requiring fearful employees to come to work, particularly if other alternatives (like telecommuting) are available.
OSHA Concerns	The Occupational Safety and Health Act (OSHA) requires employers to ensure that employees are not exposed to conditions which will cause death or serious physical harm. If an infected employee with a communicable condition comes to work and spreads the virus to others, the employer could potentially face OSHA violations, workers compensation claims and—in some jurisdictions—additional worker lawsuits, unless precautions are taken to lessen the threat.
Medical Privacy Concerns	Observing the health privacy regulations under the Health Insurance Portability and Accountability Act could raise new and challenging issues for employers during a pandemic. Without a clear understanding of what illnesses—or exposure to illness—an employee is obligated to disclose and an employer might communicate, employers could leave themselves wide open to privacy invasion and discrimination claims. The actions of public health authorities—critical in many respects for the nation's reaction to these important health issues—will have a bearing on reporting requirements, and potential insulation for employers.

Source: Littler Mendelson, P.C.

C.T. Hew, chairman of Hong Kong-based communications consulting firm Hew & Associates, pointed to one oversight some large companies made during the Sars crisis. Because of the sheer scale of the organization, firms decided to use the "cascading" approach, whereby communications were decentralized to managers on the frontline. While this approach can be effective under normal business conditions, it was not an appropriate method for dealing with Sars. Often these managers did not have sufficient information, but because they felt the need to have all the answers all the time, some business heads went beyond what they should have told the staff and started to "go off the page," deviating from the company line, often with devastating consequences. To counter this, Hew advised companies to have clear policies communicated through an effective communication structure. Normally this means having a centralized communications function as part of the company's pandemic crisis team. It is critical that this crisis team is competent, is trusted and respected by internal and external audiences. Companies need to bear in mind that often, how something is said can be more important than what is said, Hew added.

The means by which a company chooses to communicate to its employees is also important. As the case studies in Chapter 6 showed, many companies are using dedicated websites, normally edited by their own corporate communications teams. In the event of a flu pandemic, content for this site could be drawn from the company's pandemic advisory team and senior management and could provide regular updates and guidance in a simple format. The aim of the site would be to encourage staff to get their information from company sources rather than rely on incomplete or alarmist media reports. In the absence of sophisticated websites, companies could set up telephone hotlines instead.

Internal communication efforts should start early and have a large educational component. Informing employees on flu pandemics, hygiene practices to prevent contamination, as well as company policy on sick leave, are just some of the important communication messages that need to be sent early in the pre-pandemic phase. As mentioned, listed companies must approach external communications with extreme caution. Statements that are based on accurate and scientific information should be used to manage stakeholders' expectations. Liaising with government and local authorities will also be an important part of the communication team's tasks. In all communication, consistency is key. Ideally, critical information should be conveyed by one person, or a small group of people, preferably at regular intervals. Communication teams should also plan for scenarios where traditional means of communicating with staff and the public may not be available, and should also consider using less traditional methods to communicate with their audience such as short messages (SMS) and voicemail.

It is important not to lose sight of the real reason why communications are important—to save lives. Historian John Barry said that in 1918 the government only told half truths, including the then-US surgeon general who told the public: "You have nothing to fear if you take the proper precautions." But scant information was given as to what those precautions were. In a few places where authorities were more open and gave citizens explicit instructions on wearing protective face masks, such as in San Francisco, honesty paid off, Barry said. Even though the city was hit hard by Spanish flu, it did not experience the same degree of social breakdown that was seen elsewhere in the US.

5. Health issues:
At the core of any company's business continuity plan for a flu pandemic is, of course, the health and welfare of employees, customers, suppliers and business partners. This concern should drive all elements of the plan. As such it should not be considered as

a standalone factor. Even so, given the importance of the topic, this section will touch on some of the main activities a "reasonable" company might be expected to incorporate into its pandemic plan.

Many companies are encouraging employees to get vaccinated against seasonal flu, with some firms offering subsidized vaccinations. Companies say they offer this service because it constitutes good corporate citizenship in terms of promoting general community health. In addition, providing such a service could reduce the opportunity for flu viruses to mutate and could help doctors by screening out seasonal flu from pandemic flu. Whatever the real effect of these measures, they can act as an important psychological boost to the sense of security among employees.

An even more controversial question is whether a company should stockpile Tamiflu or any other antiviral drugs. In general, the conventional practice at most companies is *not* to stockpile the drug. Often this is in response to subtle appeals from governments to keep sufficient supplies of the drug for prophylactic use by frontline medical workers and for people who need it most—those who contract pandemic flu.

In light of previous discussions of the potential liability of companies, if Tamiflu (or another antiviral) is available and if there is scientific evidence that shows it has at least some potential to be effective against the pandemic, then surely a "reasonable" company might be expected to stockpile. If a company decides against stockpiling, then it should document its rationale. Vague considerations such as "government officials' encouragement not to stockpile" may not be sufficient post-pandemic when a very different political climate might emerge.

Foster from Hill & Associates said the issue of antivirals is not straightforward.

"There are complex legal and moral issues here," he said. "Tamiflu is a prescribed drug. Stockpiling may lead to misuse and wastage."

Foster said that in any case, international organizations and governments are expected to sequester stockpiles in the event of a pandemic.

Other more easily addressed considerations include the need to stockpile supplies of face masks, alcohol swipes and personal protective equipment (PPE). Educating employees on personal hygiene is a basic but often overlooked activity. It is advisable to err on the side of caution: for example, it should not be assumed that everyone can tell the difference between influenza and a cold, or that employees know proper hand-washing techniques.

Social distancing measures are also key: large gatherings should be kept to a minimum, and tele- and videoconferencing encouraged. Contact tracing was an important tool in the fight against Sars. This involved identifying the people who had come into contact with an infected person in the period immediately prior to contamination. Once successfully tracked down, these people were usually quarantined with the aim of stopping the spread of the mysterious disease in its tracks. The approach, which was relatively effective with Sars, may not be so useful under a pandemic flu scenario. Flu can take several days before its symptoms show. This increases the difficulty of contact tracing. Even so, a company should prepare for the possibility of having to conduct contact tracing. This entails ensuring that there is a comprehensive database of employee contact details, including the contact numbers for the employee's family. International organizations with operations in several countries will face the added complication of having to trace contacts in different languages.

This is hardly an exhaustive list of what a company might be expected to do to look after employee health and welfare. Similar precautions also need to be extended to customers, suppliers, business partners and visitors. Given that health issues are central to an effective continuity plan for pandemics, companies can stand to benefit by seeking external support and advice from medical professionals.

6. Business Goals

One aspect that is often overlooked in business continuity planning for pandemics is: what about financial goals? If demand and productivity plummet, revenues and profits will do the same. Failing to meet earning projections will have serious consequences, especially for listed companies.

As IMA Asia analyst Richard Martin observed, there may come a point when a company has to abandon its normal business goals (financial, market share, production, quality, etc.) and switch to "crisis business goals." Similarly, once the pandemic has abated, companies may wish to set "recovery business goals."[5]

The degree to which crisis goals differ from normal goals or recovery goals will depend on the extent to which the pandemic affects a company's operating environment. The important point here is that the pandemic planning team identifies trigger points for when corporate goals may need to be changed, and incorporates them into the plan. This will also help the communications team to manage shareholder and market expectations in the period immediately leading up to the announcement of new goals.

Tailoring the BCP

There is no one-size-fits-all continuity plan for a pandemic scenario. Companies should tailor a plan that best fits their corporate culture, size, the resources available, regulatory environment and the characteristics of the industry in which it competes. While it is impossible to single out the areas that need special attention for every single sector of the economy, the following examples are meant to highlight how pandemic plans for different industries will need to pay special attention to certain elements of their businesses.

Nowhere is this more obvious than in the case of the healthcare industry which will be at the frontline of any pandemic flu crisis, mild or severe. Unlike other industries, hospital employees will come into contact with pandemic flu as a core part of their jobs. This means that protecting frontline doctors and nurses as well as support staff from infection will be critical. With medical care, the option of working from home does not exist. In order to minimize this risk, PPE will be a critical weapon in keeping healthcare workers healthy. Scientists at the Hong Kong Polytechnic University have conducted research into different types of PPE and concluded that the choice of the right PPE is critical to ensure that healthcare workers are comfortable carrying out their tasks, and recommended different types of PPE to be worn depending on the task performed. More importantly, hospital management needs to make sure it has sufficient supplies of PPE to last over the period of a pandemic.[6] Failure to secure enough supplies could seriously jeopardize efficient treatment as healthcare workers refuse to report for duty.

The same can be said for antiviral drugs stockpiles. Enough supplies of Tamiflu and Relenza should be made available for prophylactic use by hospital staff. Hospital management will need to secure ample supplies of essential medications for patient treatment, including antiviral drugs and antibiotics to treat secondary infections that may accompany pandemic flu.

Should a severe pandemic hit, then hospitals will most likely be thrown into chaos. In 1918, health workers were so overwhelmed that authorities had to make a plea for volunteers in order to deal with the acute shortage of medical professionals, especially nurses. If the number of patients seeking treatment and/or infection rates are exceptionally high, then hospitals need to consider how they might handle such a situation, and whether implementing a home-visit system would be feasible.

Staffing capacity, as well as physical capacity limitations of hospitals, are two areas that will require close attention from pandemic planning teams in the healthcare industry. Planners should also consider freeing up hospital bed capacity by defining in advance what types of surgery and other medical interventions will not be performed during the peak of a pandemic crisis.

Companies in the IT industry will see a huge demand for their services as clients that have failed to plan appropriately scramble to upgrade computer systems and rush to get employees set up with the right tools to conduct work from home. Computer manufacturers need to pay special attention in their plans to supply chain issues and might want to consider developing a portfolio of alternative suppliers and logistics providers to minimize disruption. On-site technical support would probably need to be significantly curtailed during a pandemic, so planning should include provisions for greater technical support offerings either through the internet or expanded call centers. Again, human resources and skill constraints will need to be addressed.

The CBO predicted that the impact on the agricultural sector in the US would be less than on any other sector in the economy, at least in terms of demand for produce. Absenteeism in this sector is also expected to be lower than in other industries due in part to the relative isolation of farm workers compared to employees of corporations in large urban areas. However, that does not change the fact that companies operating in this sector will also need pandemic plans which factor in the special considerations of this vital area of the economy. Points that merit special attention include compliance with tighter government regulation of animal husbandry practices. Food manufacturers should plan for disruption to supply chains. They should also expect to have to work closely with the authorities since the supply of food to the community will become a major priority for state and local governments around the world.

These are just some examples of how different industries will need to adapt or focus their pandemic plans to reflect the nature of their business and the product or service they provide. The pandemic planning team for every company needs to consider these factors carefully and tailor the business continuity plan accordingly. In this respect industry associations can play an important role by bringing member companies together to brainstorm issues that are specific to their industry.

Rehearsing, Activating and Reactivating the BCP

A good business continuity plan should withstand rigorous testing during the rehearsal stage. "Role play and table top management team training highlights the weaknesses and allows management to visualize their specific roles and responsibilities," said Foster.

Finally, the pandemic plan should contain special details of precisely when different stages of the plan should be implemented. These trigger points can be independently decided by companies or can be linked to an external organization's pandemic alert code. One approach would be to line up trigger points with the WHO's alert codes (see chart). The New Zealand government has gone one step further and has issued a list of suggested actions businesses can take for each level of New Zealand's pandemic alert code (see Table 7). Given that a pandemic can be expected to come in waves, companies should be prepared to have to reactivate their plans as the pandemic may come in different waves.

WHO Global Pandemic Phases
WHO has currently identified six specific phases that would cover the generation of a pandemic:

Inter-pandemic period
Phase 1:   No new influenza subtypes have been detected in humans. An influenza virus subtype that has caused human infection may be present in animals. The risk of human infection is considered to be low.

Phase 2:   No new influenza virus subtypes have been detected in humans. However, a circulating animal influenza virus subtype poses a substantial risk of human disease.

Pandemic alert period
Phase 3:   Human infection(s) with a new subtype are reported. There are no instances of human-to-human spread, or at most, rare instances of spread to a close contact.

Phase 4:   Small cluster(s), meaning less than 25 people, lasting less than two weeks, with limited human-to-human transmission occur, but spread is still highly localized, suggesting that the virus is not well adapted to humans.

Phase 5:   Larger cluster(s), meaning between 25-50 people, lasting from two to four weeks, appear. While human-to-human transmission is still localized, the virus appears to be increasingly better adapted to humans. Though it is not yet fully transmissible, there is a substantial pandemic risk.

Pandemic period
Phase 6:   Virus transmission increases significantly and there is sustained transmissibility in the general population.

Source: WHO Handbook for Journalists: Influenza Pandemic, page 10. Updated December 2005.

Revising the pandemic level (up or down) requires that WHO consults a board of external experts to review all available data. The board will then make a recommendation to the WHO director-general, who will then decide whether the pandemic level should be changed.

Conclusions

Devising a business continuity plan for surviving a flu pandemic may seem daunting. But the reality is that there is not much choice. If companies want to be able to demonstrate post-pandemic that they acted appropriately and rationally before and during the flu pandemic, then a business continuity plan is the best place to start. But the value of a plan is more than just that. If properly executed it could save employees' lives and secure the long-term survival of the business.

Table 7: Suggested Summary Actions for Businesses during each Alert Code

Stage	New Zealand Strategy	Ministry of Health/ District Health Board Alert Code	Suggested Actions for Business
1	Plan for it (Planning)	WHITE (Information/ advisory)	Review business continuity plans: • Identify essential services (including contractors), facilities/plants, other production inputs • Plan for up to 50% staff absences for periods of 2-3 weeks at the height of the pandemic, and lower levels of staff absences for a few weeks on either side of the pandemic • Assess core staff and skill requirements, and ensure essential positions are backed-up by an alternative staff member • Identify ways to increase "social distancing" in the workplace, reduce movement, etc. • Consider organizational policies to encourage the sick to stay at home and enable staff to work from home
		YELLOW (Standby)	• Identify ways to minimize illness amongst staff and customers, and consider how essential messages (e.g. basic hygiene) can be communicated to staff • Identify needs for personal protective equipment (PPE) and cleaning equipment, and check air conditioning. Purchase additional contingency supplies

Table 7 – *cont'd*

2	Keep it out (Border Management)	RED* (Activation)	• Alert staff to change in pandemic status • Activate overseas travel restrictions • Review/test essential business continuity measures
3	Stamp it out (Cluster control)		• Alert staff to change in pandemic status • Activate essential business continuity measures • Activate measures to minimize introduction and/or spread of influenza in work place (post notices, social distancing; managing ill staff members, workplace cleaning, etc. • Communicate with staff to promote confidence in the workplace • Activate contact tracing where staff become ill at work during Cluster Control phase • Activate process for recovered/ well staff members to return to work
4	Manage it (Pandemic Management)		
5	Recover from it (Recovery)	GREEN (Stand down)	• Manage return to business as normal

* *The transition from Code White to Red could be quite quick (i.e., Code Yellow phase could be short).*

Source: Influenza Pandemic Planning: Business Continuity Planning Guide, Ministry of Economic Development, New Zealand, October 2005.© Crown Copyright.

Endnotes

1   "Managing Bird Flu: Pandemic Business Continuity Plans," Richard Martin, Asian Issues Management Paper, January 2006 issued by International Market Assessment Asia Pty. Ltd.

2   "Avian Flu: Facing the Facts, Managing the Impact, Survey Measures: Preparedness for Avian Influenza," American Chamber of Commerce, Hong Kong, January 2006

3   "Business Preparations for Pandemic Flu," Deloitte Center for Health Solutions, (2006)

4   "Managing Bird Flu: Pandemic Business Continuity Plans," Richard Martin, Asian Issues Management Paper, January 2006 issued by International Market Assessment Asia Pty. Ltd.

5   "Personal Protective Equipment: Sensing the Fit;" Professor Joanne Chung; Dr. Anthony Wong, Professor Thomas Wong, Professor Y. Li. Presentation to press, January 2006

Chapter Seven

Disaster Averted?

What happens if the pandemic flu never occurs, will all of this planning be in vain? Of course the philosophical answer to that is no, that planning is never a waste— that the time, effort and energy expended on creating a business continuity plan do not go to waste in the long run. Whether this long-term line of reasoning will fly with short-term focused investors, however, is another matter. From a practical business standpoint, there is also the chance that a company may lose credibility in the eyes of its employees, suppliers and business partners if it kicks up a big fuss about a pandemic flu that never materializes.

But the catastrophic costs embedded in the scenarios of death and economic chaos described earlier are more than adequate to justify the relatively moderate expense of developing a continuity plan to mitigate the effects of the potential disaster.

Of course, crying wolf entails its own set of perils. If a pandemic doesn't materialize, it could mean that when another threat to the world occurs, people will be less willing to listen. That is why we need to demonstrate that taking preventative action on avian flu now is based on sound reasoning and a very real threat.

Clearly, some final questions need to be addressed: will modern medicine step in and save the day with some wonder drug or vaccine that will mitigate the threat of pandemic flu? Alternatively, will there be significant improvements in animal husbandry practices around the world that will keep avian flu where it belongs: among wild birds? Or, better still, a vaccine that will eradicate the flu from birds and animals once and for all?

Unfortunately, none of these are realistic scenarios in the short-term. Nobody can say if and when the virus will mutate and begin to attack humans, but it is fair to assume that the bird flu will continue to pose a threat to wild birds and poultry for years to come. As long as H5N1 exists, the risk of a deadly outbreak implores us to be prepared for the worst.

Down on the Farm

The best way to temper the threat of avian flu is to make sure that any outbreaks are dealt with swiftly and thoroughly through mass culling of chickens. Better still, make sure that outbreaks don't occur in the first place by implementing heightened biosecurity measures such as not allowing farm chickens to mix with other poultry—especially wild ducks and geese. Taken together with the promotion of more hygienic wet market practices, these measures would go a long way to reducing the risk of pandemic human-to-human transmission of the flu.

At least this might have been the case if we had acted earlier. Now, it seems, it is too late, as the disease is endemic in several Southeast Asian countries. Even if we were still on time to catch the disease, the chances of getting all governments and farmers to fully implement all the recommended animal husbandry practices would be very slim. In addition to being costly, changing farming practices in such a fundamental way would have a huge social and cultural impact, and most probably would take years if not decades to fully implement.

Not surprising then that governments and scientists around the world have come to the realization that if they want to protect human beings from pandemic influenza, medicine in the form of vaccines and antiviral drugs are their best option. Yet using medication to prevent transmission of the disease or to weaken it in some way is by no means a quick fix to the problem. The road to developing a vaccine is long and bumpy and entails its own set of dangers.

Difficult Diagnoses

Before examining what the world of medicine might have in store for avian influenza, it's worth considering the issue of diagnosis.

For an antiviral drug to be effective it has, of course, to be given to the right patient. In other words, doctors and nurses must be able to recognize when a patient is suffering from pandemic flu. Many poorer countries under threat from avian influenza desperately lack any semblance of the healthcare infrastructure needed to properly identify patients suffering from the disease. Not only must the correct diagnosis be made, it must be made quickly if most antiviral treatments are to be effective. This is especially true of Tamiflu, which must be administered within 48 hours of the first emergence of avian flu symptoms.

In Thailand, in a case where a mother and her daughter died of bird flu within 10 days of each other in September 2004, the 11-year-old daughter was originally diagnosed as having dengue fever. These mistaken diagnoses mean that patients will be treated incorrectly, giving the virus more time to spread.

Earlier, we saw how a model developed by one group of scientists asserts that a pandemic could be stopped provided that the point of the outbreak is identified early and that the location in question is flooded with antiviral drugs.

While it is true that extended media coverage of bird flu together with government campaigns have succeeded in increasing awareness of the disease even in rural farming areas, these programs have only managed to scratch the surface, and once the media attention subsides, farmers and doctors alike will turn their minds to other, more immediately pressing matters.

For sure, any advancement in vaccine development should be greeted with cheers, and moves to increase antiviral drug stockpiles welcomed. However, it is important to remember that medicines will only be effective insofar as affected countries have a suitably developed healthcare system, both to diagnose and care for the sick, and to administer the drugs and vaccines.

In Tamiflu We Trust?

While some progress has been made in the race for a vaccine against avian flu, for now, the only medications with some degree of proven efficacy are antiviral drugs. But even here, there are some serious doubts emerging as to how effective they can really be in the event of a flu pandemic.

Two main types of antiviral drugs can be used against influenza in general. The first type, the so-called "M2 inhibitors"—amantadine and rimantadine—have been around for ages. They are affordable and have a long shelf-life. Too bad, then, that they do not work against the H5N1.

The second group of antiviral drugs are the neuraminidase inhibitors, which includes oseltamivir (Tamiflu) and zanamivir (Relenza). Tamiflu—developed by Swiss pharmaceutical company Roche Holding AG—is the most well-known in this group. The two main drawbacks for the neuraminidase inhibitors are their high price and very limited supply. Even more alarming, serious concerns have emerged recently about the effectiveness of these drugs. A study published in January 2006 in the *Lancet*[1] medical journal states that while they may reduce symptoms of the flu, there is no evidence that neuraminidase inhibitors actually combat the H5N1 virus.

Further, researchers note that strains of the virus seem to be developing resistance to neuraminidase inhibitors: in Vietnam, eight of the 10 people infected with avian flu and treated with the drug died.

Questions about the efficacy of these drugs aside, supply constraints remain considerable, despite plans by the manufacturer to expand production capacity. The limited production capacity for Tamiflu coupled with the soaring demand from governments and consumers around the world for the drug suggests that—unless there is a significant increase in production capacity—it will remain at its prohibitively expensive price of just under $4 a capsule. This implies that a normal course of treatment of 10 capsules could cost as much as $40 per person—well beyond the reach of many in developing countries.

Part of the problem is that the drug has no significant competitor in the market. The alternative, Relenza, manufactured by British pharmaceutical company GlaxoSmithKline, is not as popular as Tamiflu since it can only be taken via an inhaler, rendering it more difficult to administer. Roche is rumored to be expanding production capacity for the drug by building a new plant in the US. No timeline has been given for this, however, and it could be several years before a new facility becomes fully operational.

In the meantime, the developed nations of the world are not put off by the high prices. *The Wall Street Journal*[2] reports that, taken together, Australia, New Zealand, France, Norway and Finland have placed orders for tens of millions of Tamiflu treatments, while in the US, President George W. Bush has announced a plan to build enough stockpiles of the drug to treat one in four Americans, assuming an infection rate of 25% of the population.

Other caveats about antivirals: They must be administered within a short period of diagnosis (48 hours in the case of Tamiflu) and they have a relatively limited shelf-life. This means that the billions of dollars that governments around the world are spending to buy and stock the drug, could end up being money down the drain as authorities are forced to dump out-of-date inventories of the drug.

Still, in the absence of a vaccine, antiviral drugs remain the only option. If it functions properly, it should help dampen the impact of an avian flu outbreak, while taking it for prophylactic purposes will allow medical workers to tend to the sick with reduced risk of contamination. As such, antiviral drugs allow us to buy time—albeit with a hefty price tag. Some experts said that its use could provide a buffer of six months, just about enough time for scientists to develop a suitable vaccine.

The Quest for the Elusive Vaccine

On August 6, 2005, scientists in the US announced a significant breakthrough in the ongoing search for a vaccine against avian influenza. For the first time since the first outbreaks of the current wave of the disease were reported in 2003, tests of a human vaccine yielded positive results from test subjects. Even though the vaccine still has to undergo clinical trials, production has begun with an initial aim of manufacturing eight million doses.[3]

Yet there are several reasons why the world cannot afford to be complacent at this point. For one, the track record for producing seasonal vaccines against influenza has been abysmal. Each year, vaccines are produced to ward off traditional or seasonal influenza. Yet mishandling and contamination during the vaccine preparation period at production plants have repeatedly had adverse effects on global production. In July 2005, biotech company Chiron revealed that, as a result of bacterial contamination at one of its plants in Germany, it would be unable to produce or market any vaccine for the entire year of 2005. Just 10 months before, the same company had to halt production of flu vaccines earmarked for the US market due to contamination by a bacterium called serratia, this time at its plant in Liverpool, England. *The Wall Street Journal*[4] estimated that the shutdown cut the supply of flu vaccines to the US market by half.

No doubt factors specific to Chiron were involved in both incidents; other firms such as Sanofi Pasteur have had greater success in vaccine production. What's important to note here is that making a vaccine for the influenza virus is not a simple process to be undertaken in haste, and that the potential for production to be severely hampered due to contamination is significantly high. With the manufacture of these drugs concentrated into just a few locations, an accident at one factory has a marked impact on global supply.

It is also worth noting that the US scientists who achieved the vaccine breakthrough did so by using levels of antigens six times the normal amount used in seasonal flu treatments. An antigen is a substance that, when introduced into the body, produces an antibody, which gives rise to an immune response. The trouble is that antigen material is very scarce. This means that large-scale production of a vaccine that uses such high levels of antigens will be extremely challenging.

Yet these problems are insignificant in comparison to some of the other obstacles that lie in wait for scientists. When developing a flu vaccine, scientists first need to examine the flu virus, and identify the strains that are unique to it. Only when they have these parts— known as isolates—can they begin the process of producing a vaccine. This is tricky since isolates are highly prone to contamination and producing large quantities of flu vaccine using existing technologies is notoriously time consuming. Needless to say, biotech firms could stand to waste millions of dollars without ever successfully producing an effective vaccine.

In the case of avian influenza, these risks are even higher. This is because the virus is particularly prone to mutation and is highly pathogenic. Mutation is one of the reasons why some experts greeted the announcement of the generation of a vaccine by US researchers with skepticism. How can a vaccine that was developed using strains of a virus from outbreaks that occurred in Vietnam some years ago, ever hope to be effective on an avian flu outbreak that might occur one, two or maybe three or more years from now? By then the virus might have changed so significantly that the vaccine would no longer be effective.

Despite this, there is no shortage in the interest being shown by biotech firms to win the race for a bird flu vaccine for humans. In Vietnam—which until recently was the center of deadly outbreak—a host of companies from the US, the UK and Japan descended on the country. They have only one goal: to get the virus isolates and dash back to their home country to develop the vaccine.

The Great Patent Debate

It is no mystery why these companies are so driven in their quest. As P.Y. Leung of Hong Kong's CHP explained: "…the people who have the vaccine are going to be able to recover economically more quickly."

By producing the vaccine at home, countries can protect their own populations without relying on supply from abroad. In addition, the price of the drug can be set sufficiently high in order for companies to recoup the costs of research and development, and maybe even make a profit.

For Roche, soaring demand for its antiviral drugs have translated into billions of dollars in additional revenue. Some questions about the propriety of such potentially massive profits being made on the back of developing nations have lingered, and recent fears that

Roche will not be able to satisfy demand for the drug have led several Asian nations to publicly ponder the possibility of breaking Roche's patent. Pharmaceutical companies in India as well as the government of Thailand have said outright that they plan to move forward with the production of a generic form of Tamiflu, despite protestations from Roche. (Roche subsequently allowed Thailand, Indonesia and the Philippines, to make generic variations of the drug.)

A 2001 addendum to the World Trade Organization's Trade-Related Intellectual Property Rights (TRIPS) agreement allows that protecting public health is more important than intellectual property rights, and includes a provision for "compulsory licenses" to be issued when the current supply of drugs is unaffordable or inadequate to treat an epidemic or other public health emergency. This has been invoked most notably in the case of HIV medications being produced in India and distributed in developing nations with large infected populations. Proponents of compulsory licensing of Tamiflu argue that the threat from the H5N1 virus sufficiently meets the new standards set forth in the Doha Agreement. Roche insisted that it will be able to meet and even surpass global demand for the drug by 2007.

The pro-generic camp's argument is simple: protecting human life supersedes economic considerations.

Like most companies, pharmaceutical companies make decisions about the most efficient way to allocate their resources based on their expectations of future returns. The development of a drug such as Tamiflu involves the investment of millions of dollars, years of research and countless tests and trials before it ever finds its way to the shelf at your local pharmacy. Also factored into the equation are the massive liability claims that drug companies will face should something go horribly wrong when the drug is administered to humans. All of this investment and risk is undertaken with the expectation that the final product will yield sales revenue to cover all of these expenses and make a profit. Ignoring intellectual property rights could be the beginning of a slippery slope, where pharmaceutical companies lose the incentive to develop new and better drugs to combat disease.

University of Hong Kong's Malik Peiris said governments have to take responsibility to move vaccine development forward at a more rapid pace, and that they should also be willing to underwrite the considerable liability risk that biotech companies will inevitably face. Peiris points to the swine flu in 1977 in the US to illustrate the risks involved in vaccination. At that time, mass vaccinations in anticipation of a swine flu pandemic resulted in some "rare" side effects in a small number of cases, some of which may not have even been related to the vaccine itself. This led to a rash of lawsuits filed by affected patients. Biotech firms trying to develop an avian flu vaccine face even greater liability risks, given that the speed under which a vaccine is developed and deployed means companies will not have the luxury of undergoing the usual battery of stringent safety tests.

On the face of it, the patent debate may not seem as important to business executives relative to the more pressing task of developing and implementing a pandemic flu plan. Nonetheless, it is a debate that is worth following closely, given that it goes to the very heart of the world's ability to develop and supply a drug that might remove the threat of pandemic flu from the planet forever.[5]

Endnotes

1   "Antivirals for influenza in healthy adults: systematic review," T. Jefferson, V. Demicheli, D. Rivetti, M. Jones, C. Di Pietrantonj, A. Rivetti, *The Lancet* - Vol. 367, Issue 9507, Jan. 28, 2006, Pages 303-313

2   "Demand, Cost for Avian-Flu Drug Could Leave Neediest With Least," by Gautam Naik and James Hookway, *The Wall Street Journal*, May 18 2005

3   For updates on these trials see http://www3.niaid.nih.gov/news/newsreleases/2006/
     avianvax3_06.htm
4   "Chiron Halts Output at German Plant, Company Further Curtails Its Production of
     Flu Vaccine," by David P. Hamilton, *The Wall Street Journal*, July 21 2005
5   See for example http://www.cdc.gov/flu/avian/gen-info/vaccines.htm

Conclusion

"In a sense, the threat of human pandemic influenza is a 'stress test' for the international community. Are we in good shape to face a potential global disaster?"

Dr. Lee Jong-Wook,
Former Director General, WHO

Human beings are a fickle bunch. Today's "hot" topic is forgotten tomorrow. What one day is billed as the world's most pressing problem is soon relegated to a small one-inch column buried deep inside newspapers. And so it might be with pandemic flu.

Already coverage of bird flu and how it might evolve into a pandemic has seen its fair share of peaks and troughs. Yet while our attention might shift readily elsewhere in the course of the months and years ahead—especially if the number of new bird flu cases tapers off—that does not mean the threat will politely go away. The fact of the matter is that the current bird-flu outbreak has already been around for almost a decade. And while it is true that it remains primarily a bird-related disease, the death toll among humans continues to creep upward. More alarmingly, the geographic reach of the disease has spread from the confines of east and Southeast Asia to the distant shores of West Africa and Northwest Europe.

Of course, the disease may very well stay with us forever, and never make that dreaded leap to becoming transmissible from human to human. And it may never spark the pandemic flu about which so much has been said and written (including this book). But if history doesn't tell us unequivocally that a flu pandemic will happen, it certainly provides some very convincing evidence.

The 1918-19 Spanish flu, the Asian flu of 1957-58, and the Hong Kong flu of 1968-69, show clearly that pandemic flus can and do happen, and that they have catastrophic consequences.

Sometimes we try to console ourselves that the later pandemics were mild and that they "only" resulted in one or two million deaths. Yet the reality is that these numbers are so enormous that it is almost impossible for most of us to truly fathom. This is not surprising given that we have become numbed by the massive death tolls of other diseases such as HIV/AIDS that have taken tens of millions of lives.

But pandemic flu is different. History tells us it doesn't discriminate (much) between young and old, rich and poor, developed or developing country. Pandemic flu spreads around the world in a matter of weeks, if not days, leaving millions dead in its path.

This book has focused on the economic impact of a flu pandemic. But even this approach fails to capture the enormous societal, cultural and psychological damage pandemic flu have demonstrated in the past.

Yet even when we focus narrowly on economic implications alone, the consequences are still unimaginable. At worst, the world economy could be cast into a global recession, the likes of which we have not seen for decades. At best, our daily lives could be thrown into disarray and our livelihoods threatened, at least temporarily. Even if the flu itself turns out to be less potent than we envisioned, the economic impact could be magnified by widespread fear and panic. This is not speculation. We need only to look at Sars to see how a disease—which with the benefit of hindsight can be said to be relatively mild—caused so much disruption to the lives of millions around the world and especially in Asia.

Clearly the stakes are high, yet we have no guarantee that the scenarios outlined in this book will ever occur. But can we afford the risk of doing nothing? That choice lies with each individual, corporation and government. But not acting is tantamount to negligence, especially since we have been given the one luxury that other generations that lived through past pandemics didn't have—time.

True, we don't have a fully working vaccine, and the effectiveness of antiviral drugs that are available is patchy, to say the least. But even so, we have had close to a decade of constant warnings and reminders in the shape of H5N1. Fortunately, the death toll to date has been modest. We have also been blessed by heavy media attention to the matter and, most importantly, to the generous coffers of increasingly aware and proactive international organizations and governments.

We can and we must act to prepare for a possible pandemic and minimize its effects on our families and businesses. Few of us will ever be in a position to discover a new vaccine against pandemic flu. And apart from taking the necessary medical precautions, there is not much many of us can do from a scientific perspective to reduce the chances of a pandemic occurring or mitigating against its effects once it happens. Instead, we need to focus on those areas where we can take effective action. As business owners, managers and employees, the most tangible thing we can do is to attempt to minimize fear levels in the face of a pandemic. A key way of doing this is to plan. Planning based on facts, leading to sensible actions that are communicated effectively throughout our organizations and partner organizations, can be our contribution to the battle against pandemic flu.

It is essential that we remember not to plan in isolation. Every effort should be made to reach out to competitors, suppliers and—

perhaps most importantly—to national and local governments, so that plans are shared and understood by related parties.

And while another type of fear—the fear of post-pandemic litigation for example—may initially spur action, it should not be the sole motivation to draw up a business continuity plan. Instead, there are a host of other, more positive reasons to take a proactive stance on pandemic planning. These include the competitive advantage gained by simply being able to continue operating during a pandemic and to recover quickly once it has passed.

With time still on our side, now seems like the perfect moment to banish fear and start planning.

Resources

International organizations

World Health Organization (WHO)

Avian Influenza Frequently Asked Questions
http://www.who.int/csr/disease/avian_influenza/avian_faqs/en/index.html

Avian Influenza Fact Sheet
http://www.who.int/mediacentre/factsheets/avian_influenza/en/index.html

Avian influenza: assessing the pandemic threat
http://www.who.int/csr/disease/influenza/WHO_CDS_2005_29/en/12

Pandemic preparedness
http://www.who.int/csr/disease/influenza/pandemic/en/index.html

Ten things you need to know about pandemic influenza
http://www.who.int/csr/disease/influenza/pandemic10things/en/index.html

WHO checklist for influenza pandemic preparedness planning
http://www.who.int/csr/resources/publications/influenza/
WHO_CDS_CSR_GIP_2005_4/en/index.html

WHO Outbreak Communication Guidelines
www.who.int/infectious-disease-news/IDdocs/whocds200528/
whocds200528en.pdf

WHO Global Influenza Program
http://www.who.int/csr/disease/influenza/en/index.html

Influenza pandemic threat: current situation
http://www.who.int/csr/disease/avian_influenza/pandemic/en/index.html

Avian influenza and the pandemic threat in Africa: risk assessment for Africa
http://www.who.int/csr/disease/avian_influenza/riskassessmentAfrica/en/
index.html

Avian influenza: food safety issues
http://www.who.int/foodsafety/micro/avian/en/index.html

WHO guidance on public health measures in countries experiencing their first outbreaks of H5N1 avian influenza
www.who.int/csr/disease/avian_influenza/guidelines/firstoutbreak/en/index.html

World Organization for Animal Health (OIE)
http://www.oie.int/downld/AVI_AI-Asia.htm

Food and Agriculture Organization (FAO)
http://www.fao.org/ag/againfo/subjects/en/health/diseases-cards/special_avian.html

The World Bank
http://www.worldbank.org/avianflu

The International Monetary Fund
http://www.imf.org/external/pubs/ft/afp/2006/eng/022806.htm

Regional organizations

European Commission (EU)
http://europa.eu.int/comm/food/animal/diseases/controlmeasures/avian/index_en.htm

The Association of Southeast Asian Nations (Asean)
http://www.aseansec.org/Avian-Flu.pdf

Asia-Pacific Economic Cooperation (APEC)
http://www.apec.org/apec/apec_groups/som_special_task_groups/health_task_force/apec_information_on.html

Governmental organizations

United States

PandemicFlu.gov
http://pandemicflu.gov/

Centers for Disease Control and Prevention (CDC)
http://www.cdc.gov/flu/avian/index.htm

National Institute of Allergy and Infectious Diseases (NIAID)
http://www.niaid.nih.gov/factsheets/flu.htm

(US) Department of Health and Human Services
http://www.hhs.gov/pandemicflu/plan/

Canada

Public Health Agency of Canada
http://www.phac-aspc.gc.ca/influenza/avian_e.html

United Kingdom

Department of Health
http://www.dh.gov.uk/PolicyAndGuidance/EmergencyPlanning/
PandemicFlu/fs/en

Hong Kong

Center for Health Protection
http://www.chp.gov.hk/

Singapore

Ministry for Health
http://www.moh.gov.sg/corp/about/faqs/illness/
details.do?cid=cat_faqs_illness_birdflu&id=8257625

Australia

Department of Health and Ageing
http://www.health.gov.au/internet/wcms/publishing.nsf/content/health-
avian_influenza-index.htm

New Zealand

Ministry of Health
http://www.moh.govt.nz/pandemicinfluenza

Ministry of Economic Development
http://www.med.govt.nz/templates/ContentTopicSummary____14451.aspx

Republic of Ireland

Department of Health and Children
http://www.dohc.ie/issues/avian_flu/

Business continuity planning related

Mercer Human Resources Consulting
http://www.mercerhr.com/avianflu

International SOS
http://www.internationalsos.com/members_home/pandemicpreparedness/

Continuity Central
http://www.continuitycentral.com/

IMA Asia (International Market Assessment Asia PTY LTD)
http://www.imaasia.com/BirdFluIMA%20Asia_Jan06.pdf

Insurance Information Institute
http://www.iii.org/media/hottopics/insurance/birdflu/

Media
The Wall Street Journal
http://online.wsj.com/public/page/avianflu.html

CNN
http://www.cnn.com/SPECIALS/2005/flu/index.html

BBC
http://www.bbc.co.uk/health/conditions/birdflu1.shtml

Others:

Center for Infectious Disease Research and Policy (CIDRAP),
University of Minnesota
http://www.cidrap.umn.edu/cidrap/content/influenza/avianflu/

The Mayo Clinic
http://www.mayoclinic.com/health/bird-flu/DS00566

National Audubon Society, Inc.
http://www.audubon.org/bird/avianflu/avianflu.htm

Influenza.com
http://www.influenza.com/

The Poultry Site
http://www.thepoultrysite.com/avianflu/bird-flu-news.asp

ProMED-Mail
http://www.promedmail.org/pls/promed/f?p=2400:1000

The WWW Virtual Library: Medicine and Health: Epidemiology
http://www.epibiostat.ucsf.edu/epidem/epidem.html

Flu Wiki
http://www.fluwikie.com/

Index

Abraham, Thomas   47, 106
absenteeism   xiv, 44, 72, 74, 83, 96, 114
activation   119
agriculture   67, 138
Air Canada   55
aircraft   63, 66, 84, 86, 87, 88
airline   x, xiii, 56, 63, 64, 65, 66, 67, 84, 85, 86, 88, 102, 103, 105
airport   12, 63, 65
Akin Gump Strauss Hauer and Field LLP   91
Albers, Alexandria   80
alcohol swipes   111
Amantadine   124
American Chamber of Commerce in Hong Kong   90, 94
Amin, Massoud Amin   72
Amtrak   73
Anderson, Roy   42
Andrew, Hugh   79
animal husbandry practices   114, 121, 122
antibiotics   16, 113
antibody   127
antigenic drift   8, 9
antigenic shift   8, 9
antigens   127
antiretroviral therapy (ART)   17
antivirals   xiv, 10, 44, 45, 46, 48, 95, 110, 125, 130
Asia   x, xi, xii, xvi, xviii, 6, 7, 11, 14, 15, 17, 22, 31, 33, 34, 39, 50, 55, 57, 59, 60, 61, 64, 65, 69, 75, 80, 82, 93, 94, 112, 120, 133, 134, 138, 140
Asian Development Bank (ADB)   57, 65
Asian financial crisis   59, 64
Asian Flu, 1957-58   xiii, 8, 27, 54, 89, 134
Association of Asia Pacific Airlines   64
attack rate   xiv, 11, 44, 45, 58, 69, 97
audio conferencing   82
Australia   93, 125, 139
Australian National University   57
Avian influenza   xi, xiii, xvi, xvii, 2, 7, 12, 13, 14, 15, 16, 18, 60, 94, 120, 123, 126, 128, 137, 138

back-office operations   77
Bangkok   45
Barry, John   109
bars   78
basic infrastructure   70
Beijing   78
Belize   91, 92
biosecurity measures   122
biotech companies   130
bird flu   xii, xvi, xvii, 13, 14, 15, 16, 22, 31, 32, 33, 36, 44, 49, 57, 63, 64, 90, 120, 122, 123, 128, 133, 141
bond markets   58
Boxing Day tsunami of 2004   64
Brahmbhatt, Milan   xviii, 57
breach of contract   105

broadband   82, 104
Bush, George W.   125
business continuity plan   x, xi, xii,
    xvi, 43, 61, 74, 77, 80, 83, 84, 93,
    94, 95, 96, 98, 99, 103, 104, 106,
    109, 120, 115, 117, 118, 121, 136
business goals   112
business results   94
business travelers   88

call centers   97, 114
Canada   55, 56, 72, 85, 139
Cathay Pacific Airways   84
Center for Health Protection,
    CHP   11, 18
Center for Infectious Disease
    Research and Policy   63, 70, 90,
    140
Center for Infectious Disease
    Research and Policy, University of
    Minnesota   63
Center for the Development of
    Technological Leader   72
Centers for Disease Control and
    Prevention (CDC)   3, 139
Central Asia   xi
central banks   59
Cheung, Tommy   14
chickens   12, 14, 15, 122
China   xi, 11, 17, 54, 56, 65
Chiron   126, 127, 131
chronic diseases   17
cinemas   47
Cisco Systems Asia Pacific   x, 82
cold   3, 4, 111
commercial implications   86
communications   xv, 29, 38, 48, 73,
    75, 78, 84, 99, 106, 108, 109, 112
complications   3, 4, 10, 68, 69

compulsory licenses   129
computer software   xiv
Congressional Budgetary Office
    (CBO)   51, 52, 53, 54, 57, 58
consumption   56
contact tracing   48, 111, 119
cooking   15
Cooper, Sherry   54
Coronavirus   2, 11
corporate citizenship   110
corporate culture   98, 112
corporate strategies   xvi
cough   4, 10, 15
crisis business goals   112
crisis team   108
critical functions   100, 101
cross-contamination   101
cross-cutting infrastructure   70, 71,
    84

data recovery   96
dedicated strategic recovery site   76
dedicated web page   81
deflation   59
Deloitte & Touche USA   94
Deloitte Center for Health
    Solutions   94, 120
demand side   53, 54
dengue fever   64, 123
disaster-response system   91
discrimination   17, 38, 107
disinfectants, disinfection   77
Doha Agreement   129
ducks   12, 13, 14, 122

earning projections   112
Earth Institute at Columbia
    University   18
East Asia   xviii, 57

electric power   70, 72, 74, 84
electricity grid   71, 72
employee contact details   111
employee interactions   101
endemic   15, 122
entertainment   xiii, 53, 55, 67
epidemic   2, 9, 17, 18, 22, 29, 38,
    45, 56, 57, 60, 64, 129
epidemiology   ix, 141
equity markets   58
Europe   xi, 21, 25, 26, 31, 37, 94,
    133
eye infection   16

face masks   109, 111
Falvey, Cheryl   91, 104
fatality rate   11, 58, 69
feces   14
felines   13
Ferguson, Neil   44
fever   xi, 4, 10, 12, 15, 23, 64, 123
financial goals   112
financial markets   xiv
Financial Times   75, 90
flight   59, 63, 84, 85, 87, 88, 103
FluAid   43, 44, 48, 97
"Flying Without Fear"
    campaign   87
food   15, 68, 78, 87, 104, 114, 115,
    138
food and Agriculture
    Organization   138
food manufacturers   114
force majeure   105
foreseeability   91, 92
Foster, Craig   ix, 94
France   125
Frankfurt   85
Frist, Bill   51

GDP - Gross Domestic
    Product   xv, 51, 53, 54, 55, 57,
    58, 60
genetic information   6, 7
geographic reach   133
Germann, Timothy   46
Germany   126
GlaxoSmithKline   125
Guangdong Province   56

H1   6
H2   6
H3   6
H5N1   xiii, xiv, xvii, 1, 6, 7, 8, 11,
    12, 13, 15, 44, 63, 64, 92, 94, 95,
    122, 124, 129, 135, 138
H9N2   7
HA   5, 6, 8
Hanoi   85
Haworth, Jeremy   75, 93
health issues   107, 109, 111
healthcare industry   113, 114
healthcare system   17, 43, 124
hemagglutinin   6
Hew, C.T.   108
Hew & Associates   108
highly pathogenic avian influenza
    (HPAI)   2, 13
hijacking   105
Hill & Associates   ix, 94, 98, 110
HIV/AIDS   17, 18, 42, 51, 134
home-visit system   114
Hong Kong   ix, x, xi, xii, xvi, 1, 5, 8,
    11, 14, 18, 41, 47, 48, 54, 55, 56,
    58, 60, 61, 63, 64, 65, 76, 77, 78,
    79, 84, 86, 87, 88, 89, 90, 94, 106,
    108, 113, 120, 128, 130, 134, 139
[Hong Kong] Civil Aviation
    Department   87

Hong Kong flu, 1968-69   xii, 8, 54, 89, 134

Hong Kong Polytechnic University   113

Hong Kong Tourism Board   56

Hong Kong Tourism Coalition   88

Hong Kong University   46, 48

Hong Kong University's School of Public Health   46

Hongkong and Shanghai Banking Corp. (HSBC)   75

Hongkong Land   x, 78, 79, 80

hospital management   113

hospitalization   43, 67

hospitals   xiv, 3, 8, 55, 87, 92, 113, 114

human   xi, xiii, xvi, xvii, 3, 6, 7, 8, 10, 11, 13, 14, 15, 18, 44, 46, 48, 60, 66, 79, 80, 81, 91, 94, 100, 101, 114, 116, 122, 123, 126, 128, 129, 133, 139, 140

human error   91

human resources   xi, 81, 101, 114, 140

Hurricane Katrina   51, 72, 104

hygiene   79, 87, 109, 111, 118

hygiene practices   109

immune systems   6

immunity   9, 10, 89

Imperial College London   44

India   94, 129

indirect costs   52

Indonesia   7, 129

industries   xiii, 53, 66, 67, 68, 69, 71, 88, 96, 113, 114, 115

industry associations   115

infection   4, 8, 16, 54, 65, 69, 96, 101, 104, 113, 116, 125

infectious communicable disease   17

inflation   59

influenza   xi, xiii, xvi, xvii, xviii, 2, 3, 5, 6, 7, 8, 9, 12, 13, 14, 15, 16, 18, 19, 42, 45, 46, 50, 52, 57, 60, 61, 64, 68, 71, 90, 94, 99, 100, 111, 116, 119, 120, 123, 124, 126, 127, 128, 130, 133, 137, 138, 141

insurance industry   89

Insurance Information Institute   89, 140

intellectual property rights   129, 130

internal communications   78

international donors   16

International Market Assessment Asia Pty.   120

internet   70, 71, 73, 76, 84, 103, 114, 139

inter-pandemic period   116

intervention techniques   49

intranet   75, 81, 86

investment   xi, 36, 48, 56, 78, 80, 104, 105, 129

investment behavior   56

investors   59, 121

isolation   45, 48, 49, 79, 114, 135

IT   73, 77, 83, 96, 114

Italy   13, 25, 26

Japan   61, 128

Jeffs, Jim   77

jet flu   87

juries   91

Kappel, Anne Marie   73

Kenya   42

Kilburn, Mike   14

Kuala Lumpur   64

labor   53, 70, 71, 72, 74, 101, 105, 107
labor laws   101, 105
labor supply   53, 70
Lancet   124, 130
Laos   45
law   42, 49, 78, 101, 102, 105, 106
Leavitt, Michael   3, 18
Lee, Jong-Wha   56, 61
Lehman Brothers   59, 60, 61
Leung, Gabriel   ix, 41, 46
Leung, P.Y.   11, 12, 18, 128
Level 3 Communications   73
liability   104, 105, 110, 129, 130
life insurance policies   89
listed companies   109, 112
Littler Mendelson   106, 107
Liverpool, England   127
logistics   53, 67, 70, 114
Longini, Ira   46
Los Angeles   85

M2 inhibitors   124
malaria   18, 64
Malaysia   64, 65
management   19, 64, 75, 78, 79, 80, 85, 87, 91, 93, 94, 95, 98, 108, 113, 115, 119, 120
managers   xvii, 48, 70, 78, 81, 83, 84, 86, 98, 102, 108, 135
market expectations   112
Martin, Richard   11, 93, 112, 120
mathematical models   42, 46
McKibbin, Warwick   56
Media   47, 106, 140
media   xi, xiii, xvi, 1, 2, 24, 31, 38, 47, 48, 81, 106, 108, 123, 124, 135
medical advisors   99
Middle East   94

migratory birds   13, 14, 15
mitigate   xvii, 92, 99, 121
mitigation strategies   49
Morgan Stanley Asia   x, 80
mortality   13, 43, 44, 54, 59
mucus   14
muscle pain   10
mutating   7

N1   6
N2   6
NA   5, 6, 8
National Summit on Business Planning for Pandemic Influenza   70
natural disasters   32, 95, 100
negligence   105, 135
network infrastructure   83
Neuraminidase   5, 6
Neuraminidase inhibitors   16, 124, 125
New Orleans   51
New York   23, 25, 37, 73
New Zealand   96, 97, 99, 100, 115, 118, 119, 125, 139
news organization   xvii
newsletters   86
Northwest Europe   133
Norway   25, 125
notices   86, 119
nurses   37, 75,113, 123

Omi, Shigeru   16
operating leases   66
ornithologists   14
oseltamivir   16, 44, 124
Osterholm, Michael   70, 90
outpatients   43
Oxford University   42

pandemic alert period   116
pandemic modeling   41, 49
pandemic period   96, 116
pandemic plan   xiv, 98, 99, 110,
     112, 114, 115
pandemic planning   x, 41, 42, 55,
     93, 94, 95, 98, 99, 101, 103, 105,
     112, 114, 115, 119, 136
pandemic preparedness   18, 94, 137
Peiris, Malik   ix, 1, 35, 130
personal protective equipment   111,
     118, 120
pharmaceutical companies   7, 129,
     130
Philippines   129
physical capacity   114
Piggott, Bob   75
pneumonia and other severe
     respiratory conditions   16
policymakers   42
poultry   13, 14, 15, 31, 32, 60, 122,
     141
power outages   xv
predictive models   41
pre-pandemic planning   99
productivity   xiv, 52, 73, 112
profits   112, 128
property   78, 79, 80, 129, 130
prophylaxis   45
psychological impact   xiii, 12
public gatherings   10
public health   ix, 7, 27, 29, 32, 36,
     38, 42, 43, 44, 49,41, 46, 47, 85,
     106, 107, 129, 138, 139
public statements   74, 105

Qinghai   15
quarantine   23, 29, 37, 38, 48, 49,
     55, 63, 111

rail and logistics   67
recovery business goals   112
regulatory environment   112
rehearsing   115
Relenza   16, 44, 113, 124, 125
remote access   73, 103, 104
remote location   76, 77, 82, 103
research and development   128
restaurants   47, 55, 67, 78
retailing   xiii, 15
revenues   64, 112
Riley, Steven   48
Rimantadine   124
risk   xii, 2, 3, 10, 11, 26, 32, 34,
     44, 46, 56, 60, 73, 86, 92, 94,
     95, 99, 101, 102, 103, 106, 113,
     116, 122, 126, 128, 129, 130,
     135, 137
Roche Holding AG   124
Ross, Steven   73

Sachs, Jeffrey   18
San Francisco   109
Sanders, Marshall   73
Sanofi Pasteur   127
Schabas, Richard   xi
Science Watch   1
Scott, Dominic   82
seasonal flu   xvii, 3, 9, 10, 26, 36,
     54, 63, 75, 81, 110, 127
secondary bacterial infections   16
security   73, 82, 83, 103, 104, 110
service sector   60, 70
severe acute respiratory syndrome
     (Sars)   xi
sex workers   42
Shanghai   25, 75
Shenzhen   77, 78
shipping   25, 71, 74, 84

Siberia   14

Sidorenko, Alexandra   56, 61

simulation model   79

Singapore   x, 11, 27, 34, 37, 43, 45, 49, 54, 139

Siu, Alan   55, 61

social distancing measures   45, 111

software licenses   104

Southeast Asia   6, 7, 15, 50, 133

speed   6, 46, 64, 130

Sri Lanka   1, 51

St. Jude's Children's Research Hospital   8

stakeholders   70, 109

stockpile   xvi, 63, 110, 111, 113, 124, 125

stockpiling   45, 77, 110

Subbaraman, Rob   59, 61

subsidized vaccinations   110

supply chain   xiv, 53, 72, 98, 103, 114, 115

support staff   77, 113

swine flu   30, 31, 130

Swire Pacific   64

Switzerland   45

symptoms   4, 10, 12, 15, 16, 19, 63, 65, 86, 111, 123, 124

Taiwan   11, 54

Tamiflu   xvi, 16, 36, 44, 77, 110, 113, 123, 124, 125, 129

technology   xiv, 73, 75, 77, 81, 82, 103

telecommunications   103

Tennessee   8, 51

terror attacks of Sept. 11, 2001   64, 73

terrorism   32, 64, 83, 95, 102, 105

Thailand   33, 44, 45, 123, 129

third-party vendors   81

Toronto   54, 55

tourism   xiii, 34, 55, 56, 60, 84, 88

Tourists   88

Trade-Related Intellectual Property Rights (TRIPS)   129

transportation   53, 63, 67, 68, 70, 71, 74, 84

travel and tourism industry   60

travel policies   xvi

travel restrictions   45, 65, 102, 119

trigger points   112, 115

tsunami   51, 64, 82

Turkey   xi, 14, 33

Turnbull, David   86

United Kingdom   22, 26, 28, 30, 31, 38, 45, 139

United States Congress   16

United States National Institute of Allergy and Infectious Disease (NIAID)   7, 9, 139

University of Minnesota   63, 70, 72, 90, 140

unpaid leave   87, 101

utilities   67, 70, 71

vaccinations   75, 110, 130

vaccines   xiv, 7, 16, 28, 29, 36, 123, 124, 126, 127, 131

Vancouver   85

video-surveillance cameras   83

videoconferencing   111

Vietnam   7, 33, 85, 125, 128

virologist   1

virus   xiii, xiv, xvii, 2, 5, 6, 7, 8, 9, 13, 14, 15, 17, 18, 24, 25, 26, 27, 28, 30, 32, 33, 35, 36, 37, 39, 44, 45, 46, 59, 60, 65, 75, 92, 95, 99,

107, 116, 122, 123, 124, 125,
    127, 128, 129
voicemail messaging   83
VPNs, or virtual private
    networks   82

Wall Street Journal   xv, xviii, 19,
    125, 127, 130, 131, 140
Wall Street Journal Online   xi
Washington, DC   18, 31, 91
"We Love Hong Kong"
    campaign   88
web cast   80
website   xvii, 73, 75, 88, 98, 108
Webster, Rob   8
Weisbart, Steven   89
West Africa   133
wet markets   15, 69
WHO   5, 8, 9, 13, 15, 16, 17, 18,
    27, 28, 29, 30, 34, 37, 39, 55, 75,
    82, 86, 90, 115, 116, 117, 133

WHO Global Pandemic Phases   116
WHO's alert codes   115
Wong, Alan   84
Wong, Richard   55, 61
World Bank   xiii, xviii, 57, 61, 138
World Health Organization   xiii,
    xvii, 86, 88, 137
World Organization for Animal
    Health (OIE)   29, 138
World Shipping Council   74
World Trade Organization
    (WTO)   129
World War I   24, 26

xenophobia   38

Y2K   xiv, xv, xviii
Yardeni, Edward   xv, xviii

Z genotype   7
zanamivir   16, 44, 124